DR. NOW DIET PLAN

Achieve the Shape You've Always Desired With Dr. Nowzaradan's 1200-Calorie Diet. Tasty Low-Budget Recipes With a 30-Day Meal Plan

Perry Harlan

TABLE OF CONTENTS

INTRODUCTION

1. ABOUT DR. NOWZARADAN

In the landscape of healthcare, where medical practitioners often blend into the anonymity of white coats and sterile environments, certain figures stand out—not only for their expertise but for their distinctive approach to patient care. Dr. Younan Nowzaradan, affectionately known by many as Dr. Now, is one such figure. His name resonates beyond the operating room, reaching households through television screens and now, through the pages of this guide.

To truly appreciate the nutritional strategies laid out in this book, it's essential to delve into the background and philosophy of Dr. Nowzaradan. Born in Iran in 1944, Dr. Now embarked on a journey that would see him becoming one of the foremost experts in bariatric surgery and obesity treatment in the United States. His medical journey began at the University of Tehran, where he graduated with a Doctor of Medicine degree, laying down the foundational knowledge that would support his groundbreaking career.

Dr. Nowzaradan's migration to the United States marked the next phase of his professional journey. His residency at St. Thomas Hospital in Nashville and subsequent move to Houston further honed his skills, particularly in the complex and intricate field of bariatric surgery. It's in Houston where Dr. Nowzaradan's practice took root, eventually becoming a pivotal treatment center for those grappling with severe obesity.

What defines Dr. Now beyond his medical qualifications is his holistic and compassionate approach. He doesn't just see the physical manifestations of obesity but understands the multifaceted struggle his patients endure—psychologically, emotionally, and socially. This deeper understanding of obesity's impacts is what led him to develop tailored dietary programs aimed at not just weight loss but at improving overall quality of life.

The principle of Dr. Nowzaradan's diet plan, which underpins the guidance in this book, centers around the necessity of creating a calorie deficit while ensuring balanced nutrition. His approach is often misconstrued as merely harsh due to its strict caloric limitations. However, at its core, the diet is about enabling control over one's eating habits in a way that supports substantial, yet safe, weight loss.

The 1200-calorie diet, which has gained both notoriety and respect under Dr. Now's guidance, isn't arbitrarily chosen. It's grounded in scientific research and clinical experience, tailored to prevent nutritional deficiencies while still reducing calorie intake. This delicate balance is crucial, particularly in pre-operative and post-operative care for bariatric surgery patients, ensuring they achieve and maintain the necessary weight loss milestones without compromising their overall health.

Critics and followers alike may find this approach somewhat controversial, particularly in its application to individuals of varying weights and metabolic rates. Yet, Dr. Nowzaradan emphasizes the importance of medical supervision and customization. Each of his patient's diet plans is meticulously adjusted to their medical needs, an aspect that is sometimes lost in the broad strokes painted by popular media portrayals.

It's this personalized attention that has transformed many of his severely obese patients, who often arrive feeling defeated by past failures, into success stories. They not only lose weight but regain their mobility, enhance their quality of life, and dramatically reduce the risk of weight-related diseases. These transformations are not solely medical triumphs but personal victories against the odds, often after years of struggling with weight and related health issues.

Understanding Dr. Nowzaradan's ethos helps us grasp why adhering to the 1200-calorie diet can be a transformative experience. It's not just about following a set of rules; it's about changing how we relate to food and our bodies. It demystifies the complex interplay of calories, metabolic responses, and nutrient intake, encapsulating these in practical, manageable guidelines.

In subsequent chapters, when you explore the specific components of the diet, recipes, and meal plans, remembering Dr. Nowzaradan's foundational philosophy will be crucial. His approach is not about prescribing a quick fix but about advocating for a sustainable lifestyle change that embraces nutritional awareness and healthy eating habits.

As this journey through the diet plan unfolds, consider each piece of advice as part of a larger narrative that Dr. Nowzaradan has been building throughout his career—a narrative where every individual has the potential to reclaim control over their health, one calorie at a time. This isn't merely a diet; it's a stepping stone to a renewed, sustained engagement with health and wellness.

2. THE INSPIRATION BEHIND THIS BOOK

Every book has its genesis in a moment of spark—an intersection of personal passion and societal need. For this book, "Dr. Now Diet Plan," the spark ignited from both the profound impact of Dr. Younan Nowzaradan's work and the escalating health crisis posed by obesity across the globe.

Dr. Nowzaradan, or Dr. Now as he is commonly known, has long been at the frontline of fighting obesity, a complex chronic disease that affects millions worldwide. Working in Houston, Texas, a microcosm of America's broader struggle with obesity, Dr. Now has witnessed firsthand the trials, tribulations, and triumphs associated with weight loss. It is through his dedication to transforming lives via medical and dietary intervention that the inspiration for this book was realized. While Dr. Now's surgical expertise provides life-changing weight loss solutions, he firmly believes that the true cornerstone of sustainable health transformation is nutritional education and adherence to a balanced diet. This belief stems from observing thousands of patients who struggled not just with obesity but with numerous failed attempts at dieting based on misinformation and misconceptions. The myth that weight loss is merely about willpower and eating less perpetuates a cycle of dieting failures, leading to frustration and further health complications. In reality, successful weight loss is rooted in understanding the science of nutrition and metabolism, which is why this diet plan emphasizes education as much as it does calorie counts.

The stories of Dr. Now's patients are particularly enlightening. Consider the case of a middle-aged woman who, after years of obesity-related health issues, experienced significant weight loss and improved health outcomes through Dr. Now's guided dietary plan. Her journey underscored the potential of a structured diet plan to not only facilitate rapid weight loss but to fundamentally transform one's lifestyle and wellness.

Moreover, the overwhelming public interest in Dr. Now's approach, spurred by his television appearances, revealed a broad, eager audience seeking reliable guidance in their weight loss journeys. This audience's thirst for accessible, scientifically sound dietary advice provided an additional impetus to consolidate Dr. Now's dieting principles into a comprehensive guide.

Recognizing the broader impacts of obesity on health systems, economies, and individual lives further fueled the creation of this book. Obesity is not an isolated issue; it is intertwined with numerous chronic diseases such as diabetes, hypertension, and cardiovascular disease, all of which place immense pressure on healthcare providers and systems. By empowering readers with knowledge and practical advice, this book aims to reduce such pressures by fostering healthier individuals and communities.

The format of the book was inspired by Dr. Now's practical, no-nonsense approach to dietary management. The concerned queries and confessions of many who struggled with their diets highlighted the need for a straightforward, no-frills guide that demystifies dieting and focuses on fundamental nutritional principles. This realization steered the book's narrative to encompass both the hard facts of dietary science and the motivational stories of those who have successfully navigated their weight loss paths.

Educational outreach is another pillar of inspiration behind this work. The clarity with which Dr. Now explains the complex interactions of food, metabolism, and health outcomes resonates with a broad audience. This book aspires to extend that clarity and inspiration into readers' kitchens, living rooms, and daily routines, making the science of healthy eating as approachable and digestible as a well-prepared meal. Lastly, the personal transformations that Dr. Now has facilitated inspired not just a dietary guide, but a call to action for anyone feeling overwhelmed by the challenge of obesity.

This book is for those who have been disillusioned by diet fads and temporary solutions. It is a testament to the enduring power of solid science and sustainable, informed dietary choices. Through this book, readers are invited not just to follow a diet, but to understand it; not just to lose weight, but to gain health. This is the encapsulated vision that Dr. Nowzaradan champions— a vision that promises renewed hope and vibrant health to those who commit to embracing its principles.

3. OVERVIEW OF THE 1200-CALORIE DIET PLAN

At the heart of Dr. Nowzaradan's approach to sustainable weight management lies the 1200-Calorie Diet Plan—a strategy not just centered on calorie reduction but structured around a comprehensive understanding of nutritional balance and metabolic needs. This plan, while stringent in its caloric boundaries, is designed to spark significant weight loss without sacrificing essential nutrients.

The choice of a 1200-calorie intake is far from arbitrary. It stems from a clinical balance that Dr. Nowzaradan has found most beneficial in triggering weight loss while maintaining a manageable energy level for most adults. The key here isn't merely to limit energy intake but to ensure that every calorie consumed is packed with nutrition.

Imagine the human body as a complex engine where calories are the fuel. Not all fuel types have the same quality or efficiency. The 1200-Calorie Diet is akin to choosing a premium fuel that maximizes the engine's performance—here, the performance includes burning excess fat while supporting bodily functions and overall health.

The structure of the diet is meticulously crafted to include a balanced mix of proteins, carbohydrates, and fats, tailored to optimize weight loss and metabolic health. Proteins, vital for muscle repair and growth, are a cornerstone of each meal plan within the diet. Carbohydrates are selected carefully—favoring complex carbs, which break down slowly, providing a steadier source of energy and keeping hunger pangs at bay. Fats, often misunderstood and wrongly vilified, are included in their healthiest forms to aid nutrient absorption, brain health, and satiation.

Integrating these macronutrients effectively into a limited-calorie diet requires precision. It's not about cutting out key food groups but about making smarter choices—opting for leafy greens over starchy vegetables, choosing lean proteins like fish or chicken over processed meats, and replacing saturated fats with oils rich in unsaturated fats like olive oil.

The diet plan also pays close attention to micronutrients—vitamins and minerals that play crucial roles in everything from bone health to immunological function. Neglecting these smaller but essential components of diet can lead to deficiencies and associated health issues, counteracting the benefits of weight loss. In practical terms, the 1200-Calorie Diet is structured around regular meals and controlled portions, which help in maintaining steady blood sugar levels and avoiding the spikes and falls that can lead to cravings and overeating. Each meal is designed to be filling and nutritionally balanced, ensuring that the dieter does not feel deprived, thereby making it easier to adhere to the diet in the long term.

Moreover, this calorie limit encourages the body to use stored fat as energy, thus accelerating weight loss. However, it's crucial to note that such a diet should be undertaken under medical supervision, especially for individuals with significant health issues or those who are extremely overweight, as caloric needs can vary substantially based on factors like age, sex, and level of physical activity.

Many wonder how sustainable this diet can truly be. Herein lies the importance of transitioning from the 1200-calorie plan to a slightly more liberal caloric intake once the initial weight loss goals are reached—a transition that continues to emphasize balance and nutritional quality. This approach not only helps in maintaining the weight loss but also educates the dieter about healthy eating habits that can last a lifetime.

Success stories of those who have followed this diet are not just about the pounds shed but about the transformation in their approach to eating and health. They learn to value quality over quantity, nutritional content over caloric content, and long-term health benefits over short-lived pleasures.

4. BENEFITS OF FOLLOWING THIS DIET

Firstly, the immediate and most visible benefit of following this diet is substantial weight loss. By adhering to a caloric deficit, the body is forced to use stored fat for energy, resulting in weight reduction. For individuals suffering from obesity-related health problems, this weight loss can be life-changing. It's not just about shedding pounds; it's about reclaiming control over one's health and life. Rapid weight loss, under controlled and supervised conditions, can significantly diminish the strain on the cardiovascular system and reduce blood pressure, which in long term contributes to decreased risks of heart diseases.

Moreover, the diet's structure promotes stabilized blood sugar levels, which is especially beneficial for individuals with type 2 diabetes or those at risk of developing this condition. By moderating carbohydrate intake and emphasizing complex carbs over simple sugars, the diet helps in avoiding the sharp spikes in blood sugar that can be so damaging.

Beyond the physical health improvements, the psychological benefits of following the 1200-calorie diet are profound. Weight loss and improved physical appearance can lead to enhanced self-esteem and confidence, contributing to an overall better quality of life. The discipline and habit formation required to stick to the diet plan can also foster a greater sense of control and achievement, which positively impacts mental health and emotional well-being.

Another significant advantage of this diet is the increase in energy levels and improved bodily function. It might seem counterintuitive considering the lower calorie intake, but by reducing calorie load, the body becomes more efficient in processing food and generating energy. The removal of heavy, unhealthy foods from the diet and the inclusion of nutrient-dense options contribute to a feeling of lightness and vitality, providing the energy needed to be more active.

The diet's emphasis on high-quality protein intake ensures that muscle mass is maintained even as fat is lost. Proteins are the building blocks of muscle, and their adequate consumption is vital when it comes to preserving muscle strength and function during weight loss. This is particularly important for older adults for whom muscle wastage can be a significant concern.

Further, a well-managed caloric restriction, as seen in the 1200-calorie diet, can lead to enhanced longevity and slowing down of the aging process. Research suggests that lower-calorie intake with adequate nutrition can help slow down the cellular aging process, potentially leading to a longer, healthier life.

The diet also plays a crucial role in promoting digestive health. By avoiding overly processed foods and high-fat diets, and instead focusing on high-fiber vegetables and fruits, whole grains, and lean proteins, the diet helps in maintaining a healthy digestive system, thereby reducing problems like bloating, constipation, and other gastrointestinal issues.

It's important to recognize that the 1200-calorie diet plan, while offering numerous benefits, is a means to learn and understand better eating patterns and choices. The goal of this diet is not just weight loss—it's to educate individuals on how to eat for health. As such, it serves as a foundational learning curve that teaches portion control, nutritional balance, and the importance of regular physical activity.

For those concerned about the potential blandness or monotony of a low-calorie diet, the rich variety of recipes and meal planning tips provided later in this book will demonstrate how maintaining a calorie-controlled diet does not mean sacrificing flavor or enjoyment of food. Lastly, navigating the social and emotional aspects of eating is also covered under this diet plan. Understanding how to manage social situations, holiday meals, and travel while sticking to a nutritional plan equips dieters with skills to maintain their dietary habits in various environments, promoting long-term adherence and success.

5. How to Use This Book

To get the most out of this guide, it's important to approach it not just as a collection of diet rules but as a comprehensive resource for creating a healthier lifestyle. Each chapter is crafted to function both independently and as a part of a coherent whole, allowing you the flexibility to navigate the content based on your immediate needs while ensuring a structured progression in your dietary education.

Begin with Understanding

Start at the beginning of the book, flowing through the introductory chapters that delve into the core of Dr. Nowzaradan's diet philosophy and the systemic reasoning behind the 1200-calorie restriction. A deep understanding of why you are making these dietary changes is crucial, as it builds the foundation for sustained commitment. This understanding will support you as you begin to implement the changes that the later chapters will guide you through.

Apply the Principles to Daily Eating

As you progress into the chapters detailing the diet plan itself, approach them with the intent to apply these principles to your daily eating habits. Each section on the dietary constituents—proteins, carbohydrates, and fats—provides not only the theoretical underpinnings but also practical advice on how to balance these in your meals.

Utilize Tools and Track Progress

Make use of the tools provided in the book such as meal planners, calorie charts, and tracking logs. These tools are designed to help you monitor your progress, understand your own body's responses to the diet, and make adjustments where necessary. Also, maintaining a log helps in establishing accountability—a key factor in the success of any diet plan.

Cook and Experiment with Recipes

When you reach the recipe sections, use them as a hands-on workshop to practice what you've learned. The recipes provided are meant to show how diverse and flavorful a calorie-controlled diet can be. They are designed to be easy to follow, with ingredients that are accessible. As you become more confident, start to experiment by making substitutions that cater to your taste and nutritional needs while adhering to the caloric guidelines.

Engage with Community and Support

Remember, dieting is often more successful when you have a support system. Engage with communities, whether local or online, of fellow readers or those who follow Dr. Nowzaradan's diet plans. Sharing experiences, challenges, and successes can provide motivation and new ideas, and also help in dealing with setbacks.

Reflect on Changes and Adapt

As you venture deeper into your diet journey, regularly reflect on the changes you've noticed in your health and well-being. Use the latter sections of the book to adapt your diet plan as you reach different milestones. The book is structured to provide advanced advice as you become more adept at managing your dietary habits.

Learn to Manage Setbacks

Finally, make sure to consult the sections that discuss common challenges and setbacks. These parts of the book are crucial for helping you understand how to navigate days when you feel like your progress is stalling, or when external circumstances make it difficult to stick to your plan. The design of this book is such that it can be revisited often. Each reading can provide new insights, reinforce existing knowledge, and help reinforce your commitment to your health goals. Whether you leaf through it to find specific pieces of information or read it end-to-end multiple times, this book is meant to be a continual companion in your journey toward a healthier lifestyle.

CHAPTER 1: GETTING STARTED WITH DR. NOWZARADAN'S 1200-CALORIE DIET

1. UNDERSTANDING YOUR STARTING POINT

When embarking on a diet, particularly one that's structured around a significant calorie reduction like Dr. Now's 1200-calorie plan, the first step isn't found in your kitchen or the grocery store aisles—it lives in your own personal reflections and assessments. Your starting point encompasses several key aspects: your current health status, your dietary habits, and your psychological readiness for change.

Knowing Your Health Status

Before adjusting your diet, it's essential to get a clear picture of your health. This doesn't mean you need a full medical examination, though consulting with a healthcare provider can certainly offer a beneficial overview of your nutritional needs and any specific health concerns. Instead, start with observing how you feel on a daily basis. Are there moments when you feel unusually fatigued? Do you find yourself out of breath after minor physical activities? These can be your initial indicators of your body's current state and what it might be lacking or getting too much of.

Reflect on Your Current Diet

Think about what a typical day of eating looks like for you. It's easy to overlook what we consume when we aren't paying strict attention. Maybe you're skipping breakfast, or perhaps afternoon snacks consist of quickly grabbed processed foods. Documenting everything you eat for a week can provide surprising insights into your habitual dietary patterns. This record isn't about judging yourself; it's about gaining an honest insight into your baseline, which will help in understanding what changes are needed and why certain dietary choices might have been hindering your health and wellness goals.

Psychological Readiness: Embracing Change

One of the most significant parts of understanding your starting point is acknowledging your psychological readiness. Change, even when beneficial, can be daunting. It requires stepping out of comfort zones, challenging long-held habits, and occasionally, facing the discomfort of the unfamiliar. Ask yourself: Are you prepared for this kind of commitment? Is your goal to lose weight aligned with a deeper motivation? Perhaps to lead a healthier life, or to be more active with your kids? Anchoring your diet to meaningful objectives can boost your determination and sustainability in the long run. The process of psychological preparation also involves setting realistic expectations. Rapid weight loss can be appealing, and while a 1200-calorie diet can offer quick results, it also demands consistency and mental resilience. Understanding that there will be challenges and days where everything doesn't go as planned is part of building a mindset geared toward long-term success.

Setting the Stage for Your Journey

Once you have a grasp on these elements, you're better equipped to begin the diet with clarity and purpose. The next steps aren't just about following a prescribed set of meals but adapting these new habits into your lifestyle that respects your body's needs, reflects your personal goals, and fits your daily realities.

2. BASICS OF THE 1200-CALORIE DIET

When you first hear "1200-calorie diet," your mind may immediately envision restrictive eating and constant hunger pangs. However, understanding the structure and reasoning behind this calorie level can transform your perspective, turning what seems like a daunting challenge into a manageable and enlightening journey toward better health.

The 1200-calorie diet, popularized by Dr. Nowzaradan in the context of pre-operative weight management, is fundamentally about creating a calorie deficit. This deficit compels your body to utilize stored fat for energy, facilitating weight loss. While the number 1200 isn't magical, it represents a calorie target low enough for many adults to achieve noticeable results, yet high enough to sustain basic bodily function and nutrient needs when chosen wisely.

The Concept of a Calorie Deficit

At its core, weight loss is governed by a simple scientific principle: you must burn more calories than you consume. This principle doesn't vary. However, the way individuals create a calorie deficit can and should vary, reflecting personal health profiles, activity levels, and metabolic needs. The 1200-calorie diet plan is designed with a built-in deficit assumed to suit a wide range of individuals, particularly when closely monitored by health professionals.

Nutrient Density is Key

The central tenant of the 1200-calorie diet is not just the count of calories but the quality of those calories. Nutrient-dense foods—rich in vitamins, minerals, fiber, and other nutrients while being relatively low in calories—are paramount to this dietary strategy. Incorporating a variety of whole foods such as lean proteins, whole grains, and abundant fruits and vegetables ensures that every calorie also brings a wealth of nutrients essential for maintaining health, energy levels, and metabolic processes.

The Role of Meal Planning

Meal planning becomes an indispensable tool under the 1200-calorie diet regime. Effective meal planning isn't just about portion control; it's about optimizing your food intake to ensure you feel full and nourished. This means thinking critically about what will be on your plate: balancing macronutrients—proteins, fats, and carbohydrates—to maximize satiety and nutritional content. Figuring out how to distribute your daily calorie allowance across meals and snacks can help manage hunger and prevent binge eating triggered by excessive hunger.

Mental Preparation for Small Portions

A common hurdle for many is the adjustment to smaller portion sizes. If you're accustomed to large meals, the 1200-calorie diet will necessitate a significant adjustment in how much you eat at any given time. Preparing mentally for this change is as crucial as adjusting physically. It helps to focus on the enhanced quality of your meals rather than the quantity. Over time, your stomach and taste buds can adjust, helping smaller portions become more satisfying.

Sustainability Through Adaptation

While Dr. Nowzaradan often prescribes this low-calorie diet in a controlled environment with intensive monitoring, the principles can be adapted for longer-term weight management. Transitioning from a strict 1200-calorie regimen to a slightly higher caloric intake might be necessary to maintain weight loss sustainably and healthily. Learning how to gradually increase calories while maintaining a balanced diet is a skill that will serve you well in maintaining your weight loss long-term.

Psychological Impact and Community Support

Embracing a diet as transformative as Dr. Nowzaradan's 1200-calorie plan is not merely about changing eating habits; it's about changing your lifestyle, which can significantly impact your psychological state. It's normal to experience days when you feel discouraged or disconnected from your goals. This is where community support becomes invaluable. Whether it's online forums, local support groups, or even friends and family, having a support network can provide encouragement and insight throughout your journey.

Handling Setbacks and Celebrating Victories

Every journey has its ups and downs, and weight loss is no exception. There will likely be days when you exceed your calorie target or succumb to cravings. Handling these setbacks with a mindset of learning and resilience can keep you on track without harboring guilt or frustration. Likewise, celebrating victories, no matter how small, can reinforce your commitment and boost your morale. Remember, the 1200-calorie diet is just one part of a multifaceted approach to weight loss and health improvement. It's a tool that, when used correctly, can lead to significant benefits, but it must be balanced with sensible exercise and genuine self-care to nurture all aspects of your health.

3. PREPARING YOUR MIND AND ENVIRONMENT

Preparing your mind for a diet is arguably as important as any meal plan. Mindset is the cornerstone of any successful diet venture. It's essential to approach this diet with a clear understanding of your motivations: are you looking to improve your overall health, enhance your physical appearance, or maybe boost your energy levels? Keeping these motivational factors at the forefront of your mind can fuel your commitment and help you persevere through tough days.

Furthermore, mental preparation involves setting realistic expectations about the dieting process. Quick results can be motivating, but true and sustainable change takes time. Accepting that setbacks are part of the journey can prevent feelings of disappointment and discouragement. Instead of viewing them as failures, treat them as learning opportunities that bring you one step closer to understanding what works best for your body.

Visualization is a powerful tool to mentally prepare for your diet. Imagine how you will feel and look as you make progress. Envisioning yourself enjoying a healthier life can be incredibly motivating and keep you aligned with your goals.

Creating a Supportive Environment

Your environment plays a pivotal role in the persistence and success of your diet. Start by assessing your kitchen. It's helpful to clear out temptations that could lead to off-plan eating. If high-calorie snacks or sugary foods are out of sight, they are more likely to be out of mind. Instead, fill your refrigerator and cabinets with healthy alternatives that align with the 1200-calorie diet plan. Stock up on fresh fruits, vegetables, lean proteins, and whole grains, so healthier choices are always within easy reach.

However, creating a supportive environment goes beyond just the kitchen. Consider the places you spend the most time, like your office or living room. Having healthy snacks on hand in these areas can help deter you from breaking your dietary goals when in a pinch.

Engaging Family and Friends

Support doesn't only come from the physical arrangement of your surroundings but also from the people around you. Share your goals with family and friends. They can serve as a critical source of encouragement and can help keep you accountable. Additionally, sharing your goals might even inspire them to make healthy changes in their own lives, creating a communal atmosphere of health and wellness.

It might also be beneficial to discuss your diet plan with them openly, especially if you live with family or roommates. This way, you can avoid situations that may pose challenges to your diet, such as having tempting foods around the house. Moreover, they can become your partners in trying new, healthy recipes or in maintaining a cleaner, more organized kitchen that supports your diet goals.

Managing Stress and Emotional Eating

Stress management is crucial while following a strict diet plan like the 1200-calorie diet. Stress can not only cause overeating but can also lead to choices that are counterproductive to your diet goals. Develop stress management techniques that do not involve food. Whether it's meditation, yoga, reading, or engaging in a hobby, finding ways to decompress effectively can help maintain your dietary course.

Recognize triggers that lead to emotional eating. By understanding these emotional states, you can develop healthier coping mechanisms that do not include turning to food for comfort. This recognition will not only aid in sticking to the diet but also help in developing a healthier relationship with food overall.

Regularly Scheduled Reflections

Finally, set aside time each week to reflect on your progress, challenges, and feelings. This can be a scheduled self-meeting where you assess what's working and what isn't, recalibrate your goals, or simply allow yourself some time to celebrate small victories. Regular reflections can reinforce your commitment to the diet and help adjust your approach based on practical experiences and emotional insights.

4. TRACKING YOUR PROGRESS

The Importance of Measurable Data

The act of tracking goes beyond simply stepping onto a scale; it's about gathering actionable data that provides insights into what adjustments might optimize your results. By regularly recording your weight, dietary intake, and even emotional well-being, you create a dataset that offers an objective overview of your journey.

Weight Tracking: More Than Just Numbers

Weigh yourself consistently, perhaps weekly, under the same conditions each time (e.g., first thing in the morning after using the restroom). However, it's crucial to remember that the scale tells only part of the story. Various factors such as fluid fluctuations, muscle gain, and hormonal changes can influence your weight at any given time. Therefore, don't get discouraged by minor setbacks or plateaus; they are natural parts of the weight loss process.

Food Diary: The Power of Awareness

Keeping a food diary can be an eye-opening experience, pushing you to be mindful of what, when, and why you eat. Documenting every meal, snack, and beverage intake makes you keenly aware of your eating habits, helping you identify patterns such as unnecessary snacking or reactive eating behaviors. Over time, this awareness can lead you to make healthier choices naturally, without feeling deprived.

For instance, you might notice that you tend to eat unhealthy foods when stressed or bored. Recognizing this pattern is the first step towards changing it—perhaps by substituting a walk or meditation for munching when those emotions strike.

Physical Activity Log: Celebrate Movement

Physical activity is a critical component of your weight loss journey. Like dietary intake, keeping an activity log helps you ensure you are getting enough exercise each week to meet your caloric deficit goals. It doesn't always have to be a structured exercise program; even daily activities like gardening, taking the stairs instead of the elevator, or a leisurely evening walk count towards your activity goals. Tracking these can boost your sense of accomplishment and encourage consistent behavior.

Emotional Journaling: Understanding the Psychological Journey

Weight loss affects more than your physique; it influences your emotional landscape as well. Keeping an emotional journal allows you to record how you feel each day about the diet, your progress, and any struggles you're facing. This practice can help identify emotional triggers for overeating and highlight times when you feel most motivated or defeated.

Utilizing Technology: Apps and Devices

In this digital age, numerous apps and devices can simplify the tracking process. Use fitness trackers to monitor physical activity, apps to log dietary and water intake, and even sleep trackers to ensure you're getting adequate rest. These tools not only automate the process, making it less tedious but also provide graphical insights and trends that are easy to interpret and act upon.

The Feedback Loop: Adjusting Your Strategy

As you gather data from various tracking methods, analyze them periodically to determine what's working and what isn't. This feedback loop is crucial for making informed decisions about your diet. You might discover, for instance, a need to adjust your calorie intake on days you exercise more or find that certain foods trigger overeating.

Celebrating Milestones

It's important to set milestones along your weight loss journey and celebrate when you reach them. These could be as simple as sticking to the diet plan for a full week without deviations, hitting a specific weight loss target, or mastering a new physical activity. Celebrating these victories reinforces positive behavior and helps sustain motivation over the long term.

CHAPTER 2: THE SCIENCE BEHIND RAPID WEIGHT LOSS

1. HOW THE 1200-CALORIE DIET WORKS

Metabolism and Weight Loss:

Metabolism involves a series of biochemical processes that our bodies use to convert food into energy. This energy isn't just for moving or thinking—it's the fuel for everything our body does, from growing hair to healing wounds. When food intake is reduced, our body is forced to find its fuel from another source: our fat stores. The careful calibration of the 1200-calorie intake is designed to prompt the body to make this switch effectively, leading to weight loss.

The Role of Macronutrients:

Understanding the roles of proteins, carbohydrates, and fats—the macronutrients—is pivotal. Each plays a specific role in not only providing energy but in sustaining basic bodily functions. Proteins, for instance, are crucial for muscle repair and growth. Carbohydrates, often vilified in diet culture, are the primary source of energy for the brain and body. Fats, too, are essential, serving not only as a dense form of energy but also as carriers for important vitamins and maintaining cell health.

The 1200-calorie plan doesn't just cap your calories; it reshapes your macronutrient intake. This reshaping ensures your body isn't just losing weight but is nourished. It focuses on high protein intake to support muscle mass, moderate carbohydrates to fuel daily activities, and essential fats to keep bodily functions ticking over efficiently.

The Importance of Micronutrients:

When following a restricted diet, the risk of micronutrient deficiencies increases. These nutrients, although required in smaller quantities, are vital to disease prevention, bone health, and the overall function of our bodies. This diet plan emphasizes the importance of nutrient-dense foods, which allow you to meet your micronutrient needs without exceeding caloric limits. Including a variety of vegetables, fruits, lean proteins, and whole grains can help cover these nutritional bases.

How the Body Burns Calories:

The body burns calories in three main ways: basal metabolic rate (BMR), digestion, and physical activity. BMR is the number of calories your body needs to perform basic life-sustaining functions like breathing and circulation. Digesting food also burns calories—a phenomenon known as the thermic effect of food. Lastly, physical activity, from walking to vigorous exercise, adds to this caloric expenditure. Why does this matter? Because understanding this helps tailor the 1200-calorie diet not just as a universal prescription, but as a personalized, adjustable tool.

For example, an individual with a naturally higher BMR may see quicker initial results from the diet, but adjustments might be necessary to maintain long-term weight loss without plateauing.

Long-term Effects on Metabolism:

A common concern with any low-calorie diet is the potential for it to lower the basal metabolic rate—making it harder to keep weight off in the long run. This diet counters this risk by recommending periodic reassessment and adjustment, ensuring that as your weight and health evolve, so does your approach to eating and nutrition. This dynamic aspect helps maintain metabolism and supports sustained weight loss.

Each person's journey on the 1200-calorie diet will look different, reflecting personal goals, lifestyles, and body responses. Perry's approach to this diet is akin to crafting a bespoke suit. It's not just about cutting calories—it's about learning how our bodies respond to different types of foods, activities, and lifestyle changes. It's about finding what helps us feel energetic, healthy, and fulfilled.

METABOLISM AND WEIGHT LOSS

Metabolism is akin to the unseen maestro of an orchestra, conducting behind the scenes to ensure that every bodily function performs harmoniously. Its role in weight loss is profound yet often misunderstood. On Dr. Nowzaradan's 1200-Calorie Diet, understanding metabolism isn't just about knowing how calories are burned; it's about learning how to fine-tune this maestro to work in our favor when it comes to shedding pounds.

Metabolism encompasses the whole range of biological processes that occur within our bodies to maintain life. Primarily, it converts the food we eat into the energy needed for everything from moving muscles to synthesizing hormones. But here's where it gets particularly interesting in the context of weight loss: the rate at which our bodies metabolize food — often referred to as the metabolic rate — can significantly determine how effectively we lose weight.

Imagine your metabolism as a furnace. In a well-maintained, efficient furnace, fuel is burned steadily and productively. Similarly, a body with a healthy metabolism efficiently converts dietary intake into energy, with less excess to be stored as fat. However, just as a furnace can falter without proper care, our metabolic rate can slow down if it's not optimally managed, making weight loss more challenging.

Enter the 1200-Calorie diet plan by Dr. Nowzaradan, designed not only to limit calorie intake but to optimize how these calories are burned. By providing a controlled amount of calories, this diet plan essentially teaches the body to more efficiently burn its fuel. This way, even at rest, the metabolic rate remains engaged, burning calories and, subsequently, fat.

Yet, the body's response to a significant reduction in calorie intake isn't always straightforward. Initially, when fewer calories are consumed, the body, sensing a reduction in available fuel, may decrease the metabolic rate in an attempt to conserve energy. It's a natural survival mechanism. This is the challenge that many encounter when starting a low-calorie diet — a plateau phase where weight loss slows down or stalls completely. Understanding and managing this response is crucial, and it's where the strategic composition of the 1200-calorie diet plays a pivotal role.

Protein, for instance, plays a critical role here. It has a high thermic effect, meaning it requires more energy for digestion compared to fats or carbohydrates. By increasing protein intake within the framework of 1200 calories, the diet can counteract the body's instinct to slow down its metabolism. This not only aids in preserving muscle mass, which itself contributes to a higher metabolic rate, but also keeps the metabolic fires burning more consistently.

Let's consider John's story, a composite of Dr. Nowzaradan's patients. When John started on the 1200-calorie plan, his initial weight loss was rapid, the pounds seemed to just melt away. But after a few weeks, the scale refused to budge. It was an alarming and frustrating plateau. Through careful recalibration of his meal plans, specifically by boosting his protein intake and integrating mild to moderate exercise to boost his energy expenditure, John was able to overcome this metabolic adaptation and continue towards his weight loss goals.

The exercise component cannot be overlooked. Physical activity is a torchbearer in elevating metabolic rate. By including regular exercise routines, even simple activities like walking or light aerobics, the metabolic rate is further stimulated, ensuring that the calorie deficit doesn't lead to a metabolic slowdown but is utilized to continually burn fat.

Hydration is another key player in the metabolic orchestra. Water, often underrated in diet plans, is vital for efficient metabolic processes. It aids in the transport of nutrients and oxygen to cells, helping the body burn the fuel more effectively. Many times, when metabolism seems to slow down, increasing water intake can help reinvigorate the body's metabolic processes.

Thus, as we navigate through the realms of diminished caloric intake, it's not just about eating less, but about strategically eating in a way that maximizes metabolic efficiency. The goal is to teach the body to adapt without compromise. This adaptation is not just for the duration of the diet but is a sustainable, lifelong transformation that recalibrates how the body processes what we eat.

THE ROLE OF MACRONUTRIENTS

Navigating the world of macronutrients can sometimes feel like cracking a complex code. Yet, understanding this balance is crucial in the realm of weight loss, especially when adhering to a structured plan like Dr. Nowzaradan's 1200-calorie diet. Contrary to popular belief, it's not just about reducing food intake but more importantly, about optimizing the right types of fuel—proteins, carbohydrates, and fats—that we give our body.

Let's delve deeper into these powerhouses of energy and see how each contributes to weight loss while ensuring that our body functions optimally.

We begin with proteins, often hailed as the building blocks of the body. They are vital not only because they support muscle repair and growth but also because they have a high thermic effect. This means that the body uses a significant amount of energy just to digest and metabolize protein. In the context of a calorie-restricted diet like the 1200-calorie plan, proteins help maintain muscle mass. This is crucial because muscle tissue burns more calories than fat tissue, even at rest. Thus, by incorporating sufficient amounts of protein, we ensure that our metabolic rate doesn't plummet, thereby aiding sustained weight loss.

However, the narrative doesn't end there. Quality of protein matters too. Lean proteins such as chicken breast, turkey, legumes, and fish not only provide high-quality protein but also contain less saturated fat, making them ideal for a diet aiming for weight loss. Imagine a scenario with Sarah, a character based on Dr. Nowzaradan's patient experiences. Initially, Sarah struggled with the protein component of her diet because she often chose processed meats that were high in fats. Once she switched to leaner cuts and incorporated plant-based proteins following the diet's guidance, she not only lost weight but also felt more energetic.

Next in the macronutrient trio are carbohydrates. While often demonized in the diet industry, carbohydrates are essential. They are the primary energy source for our brains and bodies. The key in a low-calorie diet is selecting the right kind of carbohydrates. Complex carbohydrates like whole grains, fruits, and vegetables are absorbed more slowly, thus providing sustained energy and keeping hunger at bay. These kinds of carbohydrates are also rich in fiber, which aids digestive health—a critical factor when overall food intake is reduced.

By focusing on these complex carbohydrates, the diet prevents spikes in blood sugar levels which can lead to increased hunger and overeating. This steady approach helps maintain a balanced energy intake throughout the day, simplifying the weight loss process. Imagine a day in John's life—another composite character—where he starts with oatmeal, has a mid-day snack of berries, and includes quinoa with vegetables for lunch. Such choices exemplify how the right carbohydrates can fit into a well-structured weight-loss regimen.

Lastly, we have fats. Yes, fats - often vilified yet indispensable. Fats are crucial for several bodily functions, including hormone production and nutrient absorption. The focus on the 1200-calorie diet is on healthy fats, which include polyunsaturated and monounsaturated fats found in foods like avocados, nuts, seeds, and olive oil. These fats not only help keep our cells functioning optimally but also help keep us satiated longer which can curb overeating.

In terms of metabolism, fats have a lower thermic effect compared to proteins but are more energy-dense. This means they must be carefully balanced to ensure they contribute to satiety without overshooting the caloric goals. Here's where strategic eating plays a crucial role. By incorporating moderate amounts of healthy fats and combining them with other macronutrients, we can create meals that are not only nutritious and within caloric limits but also satisfying.

To weave all these threads into a coherent narrative on the 1200-calorie diet involves more than just knowing what proteins, carbohydrates, and fats are. It's about understanding their role in our bodies, how they influence our metabolism, and how they can be balanced to aid in effective weight loss. Every meal becomes a calculated step towards a healthier self, meticulously crafted to ensure that while the caloric intake is limited, the nutritional value remains high.

This balanced approach towards macronutrients is not merely a prescription for weight loss but a blueprint for a healthier lifestyle. It's akin to learning a new language—the language of thoughtful nutrition. As our hypothetical patients, John and Sarah, navigate their daily meals, they are not just following a diet; they are making informed choices, empowered by their understanding of how what they eat impacts both their weight and their well-being. Thus, armed with the right knowledge and tools, anyone following this diet can look forward to not just losing weight but building a foundation of healthy eating habits that last a lifetime.

THE IMPORTANCE OF MICRONUTRIENTS

Understanding the importance of micronutrients in a diet, especially one as regimented as Dr. Nowzaradan's 1200-calorie plan, is akin to finding the keys to a more vibrant, healthier life. It's not just about losing weight; it's about nurturing a body that's being asked to make do with fewer calories. This isn't merely a reduction; it's strategic recalibration.

Trace Elements of Health

Micronutrients include a vast array of vitamins and minerals that support everything from bone health and blood clotting to energy production and immune function. Iron, zinc, calcium, and vitamins A, C, D, and E, to name a few, are not just supplementary; they are essential. They act as catalysts in metabolism and play an integral role in cellular function and repair. Imagine a low-calorie diet devoid of adequate micronutrients. It might yield weight loss, yes, but at the cost of one's overall health—potentially leading to deficiencies, a weakened immune system, and reduced bone density. Thus, the challenge is to ensure that every calorie not only counts but is also rich in these crucial elements.

Weaving Micronutrients into the Fabric of a Low-Calorie Diet

In the context of a 1200-calorie dietary limit, every bite, every sip becomes an opportunity to fuel the body with these necessary nutrients. The focus is on nutrient-dense foods, which pack a substantial amount of vitamins and minerals in a relatively low number of calories. Think brightly colored vegetables and fruits, lean proteins enriched with iron and B vitamins, and dairy products that deliver a punch of calcium and vitamin D.

Consider the daily journey of a hypothetical patient, Emma. For breakfast, she opts for a spinach and mushroom omelette—spinach providing iron and vitamins A and C, and eggs offering a good dose of vitamin D. Her snack might be a small orange, rich in vitamin C, coupled with a handful of almonds packed with vitamin E and healthy fats. Lunch could be a salad of mixed greens, tomatoes, and carrots, with a sprinkle of sunflower seeds, providing vitamins A, C, E, and selenium. Dinner might feature grilled salmon, a source of omega-3 fatty acids and vitamin B12, alongside a side of quinoa and steamed broccoli, which not only complements the meal with fiber but adds more vitamins and minerals.

The Role of Supplementation

While the focus is predominantly on obtaining micronutrients from foods, there are instances where diet alone might fall short. Here, supplementation can play a role. This is especially true for nutrients like vitamin D, which are difficult to obtain in adequate amounts from food sources alone and are crucial for bone health and immune function.

The decision to supplement should not be taken lightly and not without consulting a healthcare provider. The goal in using supplements is to fill nutritional gaps, not to replace the rich complexity of nutrients found in whole foods.

Illustrative Narratives and the Impact of Adequate Micronutrition

Real-life examples offer compelling narratives about the transformative effects of a micronutrient-rich diet. There's James, who after following a micronutrient-focused low-calorie plan, reported not just weight loss but also a significant increase in energy levels and a decrease in his previous afternoon fatigue. He credits this to the iron and B vitamins that corrected his prior deficiencies. Then there's Sarah, who found that including more calcium and vitamin D in her diet helped improve her bone density, something she hadn't thought possible while also losing weight. These stories underscore that micronutrients, while micro in size, are macro in their effect on health.

Long-term Perspective

This micronutrient-rich approach to the 1200-calorie diet is not just for the duration of weight loss but is a foundation for a lifetime of health. It teaches us to not just eat less, but to eat smart, choosing foods that offer the most nutritional bang for each caloric buck.

HOW THE BODY BURNS CALORIES

Our body expends energy in several different ways: through basal metabolic rates, physical activity, and the process of digesting food. This trio of energy-depleting actions intertwines intricately, each playing a pivotal role in the overarching strategy of weight loss.

The Basal Metabolic Rate (BMR)

At the core of our body's energy consumption is the basal metabolic rate, or BMR, which refers to the amount of energy, or calories, our body requires to carry out fundamental life-sustaining functions while at rest. These functions include breathing, circulating blood, regulating body temperature, and cell production. BMR accounts for about 60 to 75% of the daily calorie expenditure in a sedentary individual, making it a significant component of calorie burning.

Imagine your body as a complex factory that, even when closed down for the day, still needs energy to maintain its essential systems and prepare for the next day of production. That's your BMR. It's influenced by several factors including age, sex, genetics, body size, and muscle mass. Importantly, muscle tissue burns more calories at rest compared to fat tissue. Consequently, increasing muscle mass through appropriate diet and exercise, even while on a calorie-restricted diet plan, helps enhance BMR.

The Thermic Effect of Food (TEF)

When we eat, our body requires energy to digest, absorb, and metabolize the nutrients. This energy expenditure is known as the thermic effect of food. Although TEF only accounts for about 10% of the total daily caloric burn, it plays a crucial role, particularly in what we choose to eat. For instance, protein has a higher thermic effect compared to carbohydrates and fats, meaning the body uses more energy to process proteins. Thus, by aligning the diet to include adequate protein intake, not only are we supporting muscle maintenance but also boosting calorie burn via digestion.

Physical Activity

Beyond BMR and TEF, the calories we burn through physical activity, whether it's jogging, gardening, or even walking to the office, contribute significantly to our total energy expenditure. This segment of calorie burning is the most variable and controllable. Engaging in physical activities not only increases the number of calories burnt but also boosts metabolic rate even hours after exercise. It's a tool that empowers individuals, allowing them to influence their weight loss journey actively.

Telling Stories Through Caloric Burn

Consider the story of Michael, a theoretical amalgamation of Dr. Nowzaradan's patients, who initially struggled with his weight loss journey on the 1200-calorie diet. By understanding how his body burns calories, Michael began incorporating walks into his daily routine, not just as exercise but as part of his lifestyle—choosing to walk to stores, using stairs instead of elevators, and eventually enjoying hikes. These activities supplemented his dietary efforts by enhancing his total daily energy expenditure.

Similarly, we meet Laura, who balanced her diet with weight training to increase her muscle mass. Over time, despite the scales not showing dramatic drops, her body composition changed significantly, reducing body fat while increasing lean muscle. This not only made her stronger and more vital but also enhanced her BMR, helping her burn more calories even when at rest.

Harnessing Knowledge for Effective Weight Management

Understanding these components of calorie burning equips us with the power to make informed decisions about our diet and activity levels. For someone on a 1200-calorie diet, knowing how to strategically increase the body's calorie-burning processes through both nutritional choices and lifestyle changes can make the difference between a fleeting attempt at weight loss and sustained, long-term weight management.

LONG-TERM EFFECTS ON METABOLISM

Initially, one of the body's responses to a reduced calorie intake can be a decrease in the basal metabolic rate (BMR) — the amount of energy expended while at rest. This natural survival mechanism, designed to conserve energy during times of limited food availability, can be a hurdle in sustained weight management. However, the 1200-calorie diet, when followed with a thoughtful approach towards nutrition and physical activity, can mitigate these effects.

Adaptive Thermogenesis

When calorie intake suddenly drops, the body might interpret this as a signal of food scarcity and thus reduce the BMR to conserve energy—a phenomenon known as adaptive thermogenesis. While this can make continued weight loss challenging, the diet plan is structured to combat this by ensuring meals are well-balanced with adequate protein and essential nutrients that keep the metabolic rate more stable.

Muscle Mass and Metabolism

Often, in the pursuit of weight loss, there's a risk of losing not just fat but also muscle mass. Since muscle tissue is metabolically active—meaning it burns calories even when at rest—losing muscle can further slow down the metabolism. This where the diet's emphasis on protein intake plays a critical role. By ensuring the protein is a significant component of the diet, we aim to support muscle maintenance, even in a calorie deficit situation, helping sustain a healthier metabolic rate.

The Role of Exercise

Incorporating regular exercise into the lifestyle change encouraged by Dr. Nowzaradan's diet is pivotal. Exercise not only helps burn calories but can also counteract the potential decrease in metabolic rate over time. Resistance training, for example, is excellent for building and maintaining muscle mass, thus supporting a healthy metabolism. Likewise, aerobic exercises help improve cardiovascular health and boost metabolism temporarily post-exercise.

The story of Emma, a client, illustrates this perfectly. Initially resistant to incorporating exercise into her life, Emma started simple with walks and progressively included strength training into her routine. Over several months, not only did she continue to lose weight, but her overall energy levels and metabolic health improved significantly.

Metabolic Flexibility

Over time, metabolic flexibility — the body's ability to efficiently switch between burning carbs and fats for fuel — can be affected by prolonged calorie restriction. To foster flexibility, the diet alternates nutrient focus, ensuring the body remains adept at metabolizing different macronutrients effectively. This is particularly beneficial for long-term metabolic health, as it prevents the body from becoming overly reliant on one energy source.

Microbiome and Metabolism

Emerging research points to the gut microbiome playing a role in how our bodies metabolize food, affecting weight maintenance and overall health. A varied diet rich in fiber from vegetables, fruits, and whole grains supports a healthy gut microbiome, which in turn can have a positive impact on metabolism. Strategic incorporation of these elements in the 1200-calorie plan not only aids in immediate weight loss but also benefits long-term metabolic functions.

Sustainable Eating Habits

Ultimately, the goal of this diet plan is not just to reduce calorie intake temporarily but to establish sustainable eating habits. This involves learning to choose foods that are both nutrient-dense and satisfying, and understanding portion control — skills that assist in maintaining a healthy metabolism.

The narrative of Tom, once a participant in the 1200-calorie diet, now a proponent, sheds light on this transformation. Tom learned to replace his previous high-calorie, nutrient-poor choices with balanced meals high in nutrients. This did not just help him during his initial weight loss phase but became a way of life, helping him maintain his weight loss and health years down the line.

Monitoring and Adjustment

Continual monitoring and adjustments are essential with any long-term diet plan. As individuals lose weight, their caloric needs change. Periodic reassessment of caloric intake and macronutrient distribution can help maintain the optimal metabolic rate and prevent plateaus or unhealthy weight gain.

2. BENEFITS OF RAPID WEIGHT LOSS

There's something quite compelling about rapid weight loss. The idea that we can see significant results within a relatively short timeframe often feels very appealing. Sure, there are whispers about downsides and warnings, but the benefits, when executed properly, can far outweigh the temporary challenges. For those considering Dr. Nowzaradan's 1200-calorie diet, it's crucial to understand the potential health improvements, energy boosts, psychological and physical benefits, as well as how it can notably reduce the risk of chronic diseases.

First and foremost, rapid weight loss can lead to marked improvements in health. Many of Dr. Nowzaradan's patients come to him with comorbidities associated with obesity such as hypertension, diabetes, and high cholesterol. A structured, rapid weight loss plan, when closely monitored and properly followed, can help in improving or even reversing these conditions. By adhering to a calorie-restricted, nutrient-rich diet, patients often see a decrease in their blood sugar levels, a significant reduction in blood pressure, and improved cholesterol profiles within a short span of time. Interestingly, these changes can occur even before significant weight loss is achieved, primarily driven by immediate improvements in diet and metabolic health.

Another critical aspect of rapid weight loss is the surge in energy levels it can facilitate. It might seem counterintuitive, given the lower calorie intake, but many participants report a notable decrease in feelings of lethargy or fatigue as their bodies adjust to a more nutritional diet devoid of processed foods. The inclusion of balanced macronutrients—proteins, carbohydrates, and fats— in calculated amounts ensures that the body gradually shifts to utilizing fat stores for energy, a process that enhances overall vitality and stamina. This energy renewal is crucial, it invigorates patients, making them more active and further fueling weight loss and health benefits.

From a psychological standpoint, rapid weight loss can provide significant mental and emotional boosts. Seeing quick results can be incredibly motivating. Imagine watching the scale drop each week; it's a reinforcement that what you're doing is working. Patients frequently report improvements in their self-esteem and overall mood. Moreover, the structure of the diet plan equips individuals with a sense of control over their health, which can be profoundly empowering.

There's a ripple effect here: a stronger, more positive mindset can bolster one's commitment to sustaining lifestyle changes.

Let's talk about the impact on physical fitness. As weight decreases, the strain on bones and joints is alleviated, which can drastically enhance mobility and flexibility. Tasks that once seemed daunting or painful, such as climbing stairs or longer walks, become more manageable and, eventually, enjoyable. Enhanced mobility naturally encourages more physical activity, which in turn, perpetuates weight loss and muscle strengthening.

Lastly, rapid weight loss through a structured diet plan significantly mitigates the risk of chronic diseases linked to obesity. Heart disease, stroke, and certain types of cancers have all been associated with higher body fat percentages. Weight loss not only reduces these risks but also plays a critical role in the prevention of type 2 diabetes. For individuals who are pre-diabetic or at high risk, immediate and substantial weight reduction can be a decisive factor in never crossing into diabetic territories.

However, it's important to address concerns about the sustainability of rapid weight loss. Criticisms often center on potential yo-yo dieting or a swift return to old habits post-diet. This is where Dr. Nowzaradan's plan makes its mark. It isn't just about cutting calories; it focuses on teaching lifelong habits—portion control, understanding nutritional labels, and choosing whole foods over processed alternatives. The transition to a long-term, healthy lifestyle is integral to Dr. Now's approach, ensuring that once the weight is off, it stays off, and health improvements are maintained.

In summation, while the journey of rapid weight loss must be approached with diligence and care under professional guidance, its benefits are manifold. From better health markers to enhanced physical and mental well-being, from increased energy levels to reduced disease risks—the changes are profound and worth considering for those struggling with obesity-related health issues. Dr. Nowzaradan's diet plan isn't just a temporary fix; it's a gateway to a new chapter of life filled with vitality, health, and wellbeing. As you delve deeper into this book, keep in mind that each step in this diet plan has been crafted to guide you towards achieving not just a healthy weight but a healthier life.

HEALTH IMPROVEMENTS

Embarking on a rapid weight loss journey may seem daunting, but the health improvements associated with shedding those extra pounds can be transformative. Allow me to guide you through a tapestry of stories and solid science that underscore the myriad health benefits gained from a disciplined adherence to Dr. Nowzaradan's 1200-calorie diet.

Imagine someone like Sarah, a composite character based on multiple patient experiences. At 42, struggling with hypertension and teetering on the edge of type 2 diabetes, she felt trapped in her own body. Her wake-up call came during a routine visit to her doctor who expressed concern over her escalating health issues. At that moment, she knew something had to change.

Sarah's story mirrors those of thousands who take the decisive step toward a significant lifestyle change. By adopting a structured diet plan under medical supervision, the profound inward changes began to surface quickly. Within weeks, she noticed changes — not just in her physical appearance, but crucially, in her lab results.

First, let's discuss diabetes, a common specter that haunts those grappling with obesity. Excess body weight influences insulin resistance, a precursor to type 2 diabetes. When you begin to lose weight rapidly, especially through a calorie-controlled, nutrient-rich plan, insulin sensitivity improves, effectively lowering blood sugar levels. For many patients, this improvement means they can reduce or sometimes even discontinue their diabetes medications, with close supervision from their healthcare provider, of course. It's like turning back the clock, giving your body another chance to function without pharmaceutical aid.

Turning to hypertension, or high blood pressure, another prevalent concern, the link between excess weight and increased blood pressure is well documented. The mechanism is straightforward: extra body mass means more tissue that requires oxygen and nutrients, which necessitates your blood vessels to deliver more blood to the additional tissue, increasing the pressure on the walls of the arteries. By reducing body mass through a low-calorie diet, patients often experience a significant reduction in blood pressure. It is not uncommon for someone like Sarah to witness her blood pressure readings move from dangerously high to within normal ranges, a change that sometimes confounds even her own expectations.

Beyond diabetes and hypertension, weight loss substantially lowers cholesterol levels. Excess weight typically leads to elevated levels of bad cholesterol (LDL) and triglycerides, which are major risk factors for cardiovascular diseases. A strategic reduction in calorie intake effectively reduces these lipids. This not only diminishes your risk of heart disease but also enhances your body's ability to circulate blood more efficiently, thanks to clearer, less constricted vessels.

Moreover, obesity often leads to a fatty liver, which, unchecked, can progress to liver inflammation and cirrhosis. Weight loss can halt the progression, and in some cases, even reverse fatty liver disease. The liver begins to function more effectively, metabolizing fats better, which not only supports weight loss but also bolsters overall vitality and well-being.

One of the most immediate benefits reported, often overlooked in the broad spectrum of health improvements, is the reduction in joint pain.

Less weight means less strain on weight-bearing joints like the hips, knees, and ankles. For someone like Sarah, this manifests as the ability to walk further, engage more actively with her children, or even enjoy a leisurely bike ride — activities she might have avoided or struggled with previously due to joint discomfort.

Sleep is another critical, yet frequently underestimated aspect of health improved by weight loss. Obstructive sleep apnea, a condition exacerbated by excess weight, can significantly disrupt sleep patterns, leading to chronic fatigue and other serious health issues. However, as pounds are shed, many experience fewer interruptions in breathing during sleep, leading to more restful nights and energized days.

In weaving through Sarah's and similar patient stories, the overarching narrative emphasizes a holistic improvement in quality of life, stemming from adopting and maintaining Dr. Nowzaradan's 1200-calorie diet. Each story is a commitment to oneself, a testament to the resilience of the human spirit, and a celebration of reclaiming a healthy, vibrant life.

BOOSTING ENERGY LEVELS

Imagine rising each morning feeling light, energized, and ready to take on the day—a sharp contrast to the sluggish, heavy sensation that often accompanies excess weight. This isn't just a minor convenience but a profound transformation in everyday life that comes from following Dr. Nowzaradan's 1200-calorie diet plan. This subchapter explores how rapid weight loss can significantly boost energy levels, enhancing both physical and mental states, and why this energy increase occurs.

Many individuals struggling with weight issues report a constant feeling of lethargy. What they experience isn't just a simple tiredness but an overwhelming drain that impacts every aspect of their lives. Enter Alex, a real-life patient whose journey epitomizes the energy transformation we witness through significant, swift weight loss. Working a desk job and weighing in at over 300 pounds, Alex found climbing even a few stairs exhausting. The breaking point came when he felt too tired even during a short walk with his daughter. Determined to change, he turned to the 1200-calorie diet plan.

The initial phase of any diet can indeed leave individuals feeling temporarily more tired, as the body adjusts to decreased calorie intake. However, what happens thereafter is nothing short of remarkable. As the body starts to adapt, shedding fat and reducing the immense effort required simply to carry extra weight, the transformed metabolism begins using energy more efficiently.

The science behind this involves the metabolic shift from relying primarily on glucose for energy to a greater reliance on ketones —small molecules produced when fat is broken down.

This switch not only helps in consistently shedding pounds but also stabilizes energy levels throughout the day. Rather than the highs and lows associated with fluctuating blood sugar levels, individuals on a low-calorie, controlled-carb diet enjoy a more stable energy supply.

For Alex, the change was noticeable within weeks. The energy he gained as his body adjusted to its new fuel source enabled him to expand his physical activities. He started biking, a hobby he had abandoned in his twenties. Additionally, the lighter load he carried not only enhanced his physical movements but his sleep quality improved. Weight loss is famously effective at alleviating sleep apnea and other sleep disturbances, thus contributing to better rest and hence more daytime energy.

Moreover, the quality of nutrition plays a crucial role in this newfound vitality. Dr. Nowzaradan's diet plan emphasizes nutrient-dense foods that provide the vitamins and minerals necessary for optimal body function. These nutrients are essential for converting food into energy, a process that can be hampered by a diet filled with processed foods and high in sugar. By focusing on balanced meals filled with vegetables, lean proteins, and healthy fats, the diet ensures the body has all it needs to function at its best.

Mentally, the results of boosted energy levels are just as pronounced. With better energy, cognitive functions like focus and mental clarity are sharpened. Many patients report an enhanced ability to concentrate and that "mental fog" often clears. Alex discovered that not only was he more active, but he was also more productive at work and more present in his interactions.

The change in energy levels can sometimes feel miraculous. But there's nothing mystical about it—it's rooted deeply in the science of nutrition and physiology. The balanced approach of Dr. Nowzaradan's diet ensures that while the calories are restricted, the body's complex needs are met, fueling all its systems more effectively.

As weight continues to drop, the body becomes less burdened. Organs like the heart and lungs function more efficiently when not strained by excess fat. Every pound lost means less work for the heart, less crushing weight on the chest, and easier breathing—factors that collectively contribute to higher energy availability.

At the core of this energy transformation is also an emotional uplift. Feeling lighter, moving easier, and reclaiming active hobbies contribute substantially to emotional and psychological health, which in turn circles back to foster physical energy through improved motivation and vitality.

PSYCHOLOGICAL BENEFITS

The journey towards significant weight loss is not just a physical one; it profoundly influences the mental and emotional realms as well. For people who embark on Dr. Nowzaradan's 1200-calorie diet and experience rapid weight loss, psychological transformations often occur that are just as life-altering as the physical changes.

Take Mark, for example, a middle-aged software developer who had struggled with obesity since adolescence. His weight impacted not only his health but his self-esteem, social interactions, and overall happiness. Beneath the surface of his daily routines, Mark faced a constant battle with negative self-perception and social anxiety, which are not uncommon challenges among those dealing with significant weight issues. The decision to tackle his weight problem through rapid weight loss was about more than improving his physical health; it was a pathway to reclaim his mental and emotional well-being.

As Mark progressed through his weight loss journey, the first noticeable psychological benefit was an improvement in self-esteem. Weight often carries a stigma, and the judgment, whether overt or perceived, can lead to a significant emotional burden. As the pounds dropped, so did some of the barriers to Mark's self-confidence. He began experiencing a sense of achievement that snowballed with each milestone reached. This kind of positive feedback loop is critical; early successes in weight loss provide reassurance that one's personal efforts are paying off, reinforcing commitment to the journey.

Moreover, the connection between physical activity and psychological well-being cannot be overstated. As Mark lost weight, physical activities that had once seemed daunting or physically uncomfortable became more accessible. Exercise released endorphins, known as the body's "feel-good" chemicals, which naturally reduce perceptions of pain and trigger feelings of euphoria and general well-being. The regular endorphin rush contributed to an improved mood and, over time, helped alter his long-standing habits of inactivity—a change that supported both his weight loss efforts and mental health.

Social anxiety and isolation are other critical areas where rapid weight loss can have a transformative psychological impact. Prior to his weight loss, Mark often declined social invitations, fearing judgement or finding himself physically uncomfortable in public settings. As he shed his excess weight, Mark found that not only did social interactions become easier, but his desire to engage increased. This improvement is a common reflection among many who go through similar transformations. Being able to participate more fully in life leads to greater satisfaction and an enriched social life, which are powerful medicine for feelings of depression and anxiety.

Another aspect where psychological benefits manifest is in the realm of cognitive function. Obesity and poor diet can impair cognition, whereas losing weight and consuming a balanced diet can enhance cognitive performance. Mark noticed that his concentration and memory improved as he made nutritional changes and reduced his caloric intake. This cognitive boost is supported by research suggesting that a healthier diet and weight loss improve brain function, including sharper memory and better problem-solving abilities.

It's also crucial to address the role of psychological resilience. Weight loss is not a linear journey—there are ups and downs, plateaus, and challenges. Rapid weight loss often requires significant behavioral changes that, while initially challenging, can strengthen a person's coping and adaptive skills. Mark learned to manage disappointment and setbacks, skills that are transferable to other areas of life, reinforcing his overall psychological resilience.

The emotional freedom that comes with such a profound lifestyle change is something Mark—like many others—cherishes the most. He expressed feeling liberated from the weight of his past—both physically and emotionally. This sense of liberation often leads to exploring new interests, revisiting old hobbies, and, importantly, looking forward to the future with optimism.

While the journey of rapid weight loss is intensely personal and can be fraught with challenges, the psychological benefits—enhanced self-esteem, reduced anxiety, improved mood, better cognitive function, and increased resilience—contribute to a fuller, more enjoyable life. For Mark, as for many others, the decision to lose weight rapidly became less about the physical pounds shed and more about the emotional weight lifted. This profound psychological transformation supports not just a healthier lifestyle but a happier existence.

PHYSICAL FITNESS

In the realm of rapid weight loss, the upsurge in physical fitness resonates through every stride, stretch, and strength-training session. Witnessing your body rebound from the throes of excess weight into a state of enhanced mobility and endurance is not just invigorating—it's transformative.

Consider Jenna, a high school teacher in her late thirties who, before embarking on her weight loss journey with Dr. Nowzaradan's 1200-calorie diet, felt hindered by her own body. With each extra pound, her energy dipped, and what used to be simple tasks became strenuous. On the brink of giving up, Jenna decided to change her life, not fully aware of the profound impact this decision would have on her overall fitness and mobility.

As Jenna started to shed pounds, she immediately noticed certain improvements: ascending a flight of stairs no longer left her breathless, and keeping up with her students became less of a physical strain. This anecdotal evidence is mirrored by numerous studies underscoring how weight loss leads to increased aerobic capacity and stamina. As weight decreases, the heart does not have to work as hard to pump blood, significantly improving cardiovascular health and increasing one's ability to perform physical activities without undue fatigue.

Physical fitness, however, encompasses more than just enhanced aerobic abilities. As Jenna continued her journey, she also began including strength-training into her routine—a move encouraged for anyone undergoing significant weight loss. Muscle strength is critical not only for everyday activities but also for maintaining metabolic rate and supporting skeletal health. With reduced body weight, exercising becomes less taxing on the muscles and joints, decreasing the risk of injuries that can occur from carrying excess weight. Jenna found that as she lost weight, she not only felt--but also became--physically stronger.

The effects of weight loss on joint health cannot be overstated. Joint pain and deteriorative conditions like osteoarthritis are exacerbated by obesity, due to the excessive pressure placed on the joints by body weight. Weight loss significantly reduces this pressure, thus decreasing pain and improving joint function. This was a game changer for Jenna; she was not only able to participate more actively in physical activities but also experienced less day-to-day pain, further enhancing her quality of life.

An increase in physical fitness also paves the way for more involved forms of exercise, further bolstering one's health. Jenna, for example, found herself participating in local 5k runs—an activity previously unimaginable. This isn't just about the ability to run without gasping for air; it's about reclaiming a life filled with physical possibilities. Each run added a layer of confidence and proof of her increased fitness level.

Moreover, rapid weight loss and its resultant increase in physical activity play a vital role in improving body composition, not just in terms of fat loss but in increasing lean muscle mass. Muscle is metabolically active, so having more muscle compared to fat boosts the body's basal metabolic rate (BMR), meaning it burns more calories at rest. This not only aids in further weight loss but also in weight maintenance, creating a beneficial cycle that promotes continual health.

For many like Jenna, the journey towards physical fitness through weight loss is not linear. There are plateaus, there are days when old habits rear their heads, but the overarching trajectory remains upward and forward. Improved flexibility, better balance, and heightened endurance are all facets of fitness that she discovered and embraced as her weight decreased.

The emotional synergy with physical improvement carries profound implications. As physical boundaries expand, new horizons open in all aspects of life—be it social, professional, or personal. Jenna's journey from a sedentary lifestyle to one brimming with activity serves as a testament to the power of physical fitness gained through weight loss—a true metamorphosis from the inside out.

REDUCING THE RISK OF CHRONIC DISEASES

Embedded within discussions on weight loss are often profound narratives of rejuvenation and revival, but nowhere are the transformative outcomes of rapid weight loss more evident than in the dramatic reduction in the risk of chronic diseases.

Consider the story of Laura, a gentle and soft-spoken school librarian, whose battle with obesity brought on an onslaught of health issues that started in her early forties. High blood pressure, type 2 diabetes, and elevated cholesterol haunted her daily life, casting a shadow on her health and well-being. It wasn't until she encountered Dr. Nowzaradan's 1200-calorie diet that she realized her health trajectory could change radically and rapidly.

By sticking closely to a lower calorie, nutrient-dense diet, Laura saw an impressive turnabout in her health within a few months—a narrative not uncommon in the sphere of rapid weight loss. Metabolic conditions like diabetes and hypertension are directly influenced by one's weight. As body fat decreases, so does the prevalence and severity of these conditions. For individuals like Laura, this can mean reducing or sometimes entirely eliminating the need for medications, such as insulin or blood pressure controllers.

The science behind these changes relates closely to how the body processes and stores fat. Excess body fat, especially around the abdomen, interferes with the body's endocrine function, leading to insulin resistance—an early step toward diabetes. Rapid weight loss, facilitated by calorie control and enhanced nutrition, directly decreases body fat and immediately improves insulin sensitivity. Similar improvements can be observed with hypertension. Weight loss reduces stress on blood vessels, allowing them to relax and reduce the overall pressure—therefore decreasing the risk of heart disease and stroke, too.

Laura's doctor noted that with every pound she lost, her cholesterol levels began to trend downwards. High cholesterol, another risk factor for cardiovascular disease, often improves with dietary changes and weight loss. The liver, which processes body fats, functions more efficiently when not burdened by excess fat and an overabundance of rich, unhealthy foods. By transforming her diet, Laura was contributing to her liver's health and thereby significantly cutting down her heart disease risk.

Moreover, bringing weight to a healthy range also reduces the burden on the body's skeletal system and lowers inflammation, associated with a spectrum of chronic conditions from joint diseases to systemic ones like heart disease.

Laura found that as she lost weight, not only did her knees feel better, easing the pain of early osteoarthritis, but she also experienced fewer general aches and pains. Inflammation markers in blood tests, which her doctor monitored regularly, showed significant decreases.

This pattern of improvement extends further into possibilities of avoiding certain cancers linked to high body fat percentages. Research has shown a positive correlation between obesity and an increased risk of several types of cancer, including breast and colon cancer. Reducing body weight reduces this risk, providing a compelling argument for the pursuit of weight loss with intent and urgency. As Laura's physical health improved, so too did her mental health, demonstrating the interconnectedness of our physical and psychological states. This reduction in mental stress further perpetuates a lower risk of chronic diseases, affirming the body's holistic response to better weight management.

Each of these medical insights were not just abstract numbers to Laura but represented a reclaiming of her life and control over her health destiny. Dr. Nowzaradan's plan offered her more than a diet; it provided a roadmap away from chronic disease and towards a longer, healthier life. While rapid weight loss must be approached with careful medical guidance, the potential it brings to reduce the risk of many life-threatening diseases is undeniably profound. For Laura, and many others embracing this journey, the path isn't just about becoming lighter but about achieving a qualitative, healthful alteration in life. Each step forward in weight loss is, in fact, a step away from the risk of chronic disease and a step closer to a promise of longevity and vitality.

3. UNDERSTANDING MACRONUTRIENTS

PROTEINS: BUILDING BLOCKS OF THE BODY

Proteins are composed of amino acids, often referred to as the building blocks of proteins. These amino acids are categorized into essential and non-essential types. Essential amino acids cannot be produced by the body and hence must be obtained from your diet. Each protein type has a unique sequence of amino acids which determines its role and function in the body. This fascinating complexity is what helps your body perform at its optimum, repair itself, and grow stronger. The metabolic benefits of protein are equally impressive. Consuming protein has a higher thermic effect than fats or carbohydrates. This means that your body uses more energy to digest and metabolize proteins, which can aid in weight loss. This process not only helps in burning more calories but also stabilizes blood sugar levels, which can prevent the highs and lows that lead to cravings and snacking. In a diet like Dr. Nowzaradan's, where calorie intake is significantly restricted, ensuring efficient metabolism can enhance weight loss outcomes while preserving your health.

Furthermore, proteins are critical in maintaining muscle mass, especially important during weight loss. When calories are reduced, the body can sometimes turn to its own muscle tissue for energy. However, a higher intake of protein can safeguard muscle mass, as proteins help repair and build new muscle tissues. Maintaining muscle is crucial not only for physical strength and stability but also because muscle tissue burns more calories than fat tissue, even at rest. Preserving muscle mass thus boosts your metabolic rate, a boon for long-term weight management.

Let's not overlook the satiety factor. High-protein foods are more filling; they help regulate the hunger hormone ghrelin and increase the levels of peptide YY, a hormone that makes you feel full. These hormonal changes help curb appetite and can significantly reduce your calorie intake without making you feel deprived. In the narrative of weight loss, where every calorie counts, feeling full and satisfied can be the difference between success and setback.

However, while the virtues of proteins are undeniable, it's equally important to choose the right sources of protein. Lean meats like chicken, turkey, and fish are excellent sources because they provide the required proteins without too many additional fats. Plant-based proteins such as beans, lentils, and tofu not only offer protein but also bring along fibers and other nutrients benefiting overall health and aiding digestion, which can sometimes be sluggish in a low-calorie diet.

For anyone embarking on a low-calorie diet, the risk of nutrient deficiency must be managed carefully. Quality proteins are not only about building and repair; they also help ensure that various micronutrients are part of your diet. Foods rich in proteins often carry with them essential vitamins and minerals such as iron, magnesium, and zinc, further enhancing your nutritional intake.

Integrating sufficient protein within a 1200-calorie limit requires strategic thinking about your meals. It's about balance and distribution, ensuring that each meal contains enough protein to keep metabolism brisk and satiety high. This might mean allocating a portion of your breakfast to egg whites, adding a lean protein source to your lunch salad, and perhaps incorporating fish or a plant-based protein for dinner. What's important is maintaining diversity in your protein sources to cover the spectrum of essential amino acids and nutrients, thus rounding out your diet for comprehensive health benefits.

CARBOHYDRATES: ENERGY SOURCES

Carbohydrates, universally known as carbs, are the sugars, starches, and fibers found in fruits, grains, vegetables, and milk products. Chemically, they are composed of carbon, hydrogen, and oxygen. They are your body's most preferred energy source; think of them as your body's version of gasoline fueling a car. When you eat carbs, your body breaks them down into glucose (blood sugar), which is used to energize your cells, tissues, and organs. Any unused glucose is stored in the liver and muscles as glycogen for use when needed, like during a workout.

However, not all carbohydrates are created equally. They are typically categorized into two types: simple and complex. Simple carbohydrates consist of easy-to-digest, basic sugars with little real value for your body—often referred to as "bad" carbs. These are found in sugary drinks, desserts, and processed foods. On the other side, complex carbohydrates include fiber and starches and are packed with nutrients that are vital for your health. They are found in foods like whole grains, beans, vegetables, and fruits.

Curiously, while most weight loss narratives push for a low-carb diet, understanding the impact of carbohydrates on weight management is crucial. When you consume carbohydrates, your body releases insulin to help process the glucose in your blood. Managing this insulin response through a controlled carbohydrate intake is key to both controlling your weight and your health. Opt for complex carbohydrates—their high fiber content allows a slower release of glucose into your bloodstream, keeping blood sugar levels stable and helping you avoid the spikes and troughs associated with simple carbs.

An intriguing aspect of carbohydrates is their indirect role in weight management via satiety. Foods high in complex carbs are often rich in fiber, which doesn't make you just fuller faster; it keeps you feeling full longer. By replacing those impulse grabs for a sugary snack with more satisfying choices, maintaining a lower calorie intake becomes less of a stride against willpower and more a natural progression of a well-adjusted diet.

Concerns often arise that high-carb foods are inherently fattening. However, it's the type of carbs and the company they keep that contribute to weight gain. Processed foods high in calories and simple carbs can indeed tip the scales unfavorably. But a diet rich in fiber and whole grains can actually aid in weight loss. For instance, consider a breakfast involving steel-cut oats paired with a scatter of berries versus a bowl of sugary cereal. The former not only fuels your body better but enhances your metabolic health, too.

For those following Dr. Nowzaradan's 1200-calorie diet plan, understanding how to distribute carbohydrate intake throughout the day can amplify weight loss results. It's not just about choosing the right type of carbs but also timing their intake to support your energy levels throughout the day without overpowering your insulin response. A balanced approach—where complex carbs are tapered off through the day and complemented with adequate protein and healthy fats—can optimize both your dietary satisfaction and metabolic health.

In maneuvering through a low-calorie diet landscape, it is also prudent to address the misconception of "net carbs," which subtracts fiber from the total carbohydrates count. Understanding this can help in making informed choices about the carbs that are best for your diet plan—focusing on those that provide both energy and nutrition without empty calories.

FATS: ESSENTIAL NUTRIENTS

Fats, chemically referred to as lipids, are a diverse group of compounds essential for life. At a basic level, fats are categorized as saturated, unsaturated (which includes monounsaturated and polyunsaturated), and trans fats. Each type of fat behaves differently in our bodies and thus impacts our health in distinct ways. To harness fats beneficially in a weight loss diet, it's crucial to understand these differences.

Saturated fats are typically solid at room temperature and found in animal products such as meat and dairy, as well as some tropical oils. They can raise LDL (bad) cholesterol levels in your blood, thereby increasing the risk of heart disease and stroke. However, consuming them in moderation, as part of a balanced diet, should not be problematic.

Unsaturated fats, found in plant-based oils, nuts, seeds, and fish, are generally liquid at room temperature. These facts are considered beneficial for health as they can lower bad cholesterol levels and are heart-healthy. Especially significant in unsaturated fats are the omega-3 fatty acids, found abundantly in fish such as salmon and sardines, which are known for reducing inflammation and potentially lowering the risk of heart disease.

Trans fats are the outlier in fat types and generally should be avoided. These facts are created in an industrial process that adds hydrogen to liquid vegetable oils to make them more solid. They are found in many fried foods, baked goods, and processed snack foods. Trans fats increase bad cholesterol levels while decreasing good cholesterol levels, a double-hit for heart health.

Understanding the balance and intake of fats in a diet, especially one as restrictive as a 1200-calorie diet, is pivotal. Since fats are calorie-dense, providing 9 calories per gram compared to 4 calories per gram for both proteins and carbohydrates, they must be carefully incorporated. However, their satiety value cannot be overstated; a meal with an appropriate amount of healthy fats will help you feel fuller for longer, curbing the tendency to overeat or snack, which is vital in a calorie-limited diet. The art of integrating healthy fats into a diet plan revolves around selection and portion control.

For instance, adding a moderate amount of olive oil to a salad, eating a small portion of avocados, or including a handful of nuts in your daily intake can significantly enhance nutrient absorption, promote satiety, and support your dietary goals without exceeding your calorie limits.

Moreover, the role of fats extends beyond just satiety and calorie control. Fats are essential for the absorption of fat-soluble vitamins such as Vitamins A, D, E, and K. These vitamins are crucial for a myriad of functions in the body including but not limited to immune function, bone health, and blood clotting. In the context of a low-calorie diet, ensuring adequate fat intake means that despite limiting calorie consumption, the body does not suffer from a lack of crucial nutrients.

One of the key strategies in managing fat intake is not just selecting the right type but also distributing it properly throughout your meals. This method ensures a steady energy release, keeps hunger at bay, and optimizes metabolic health. For instance, integrating a bit of healthy fat in each meal could be part of a strategic approach to stabilize blood sugar levels and manage insulin response, both critical in a weight loss regimen.

BALANCING MACROS IN YOUR DIET

Balancing the macronutrients in your diet might sound like a scientific experiment, but it's much more akin to an art form—the art of understanding and listening to your body. In the landscape of Dr. Nowzaradan's 1200-calorie diet plan, the macronutrients—proteins, carbohydrates, and fats—play starring roles. Each one has a specific set of responsibilities that contribute to the body's well-being, and finding the right equilibrium can dramatically impact your weight loss success and overall health.

Proteins, carbohydrates, and fats each serve crucial but varying roles. Proteins rebuild tissues and act as a building block for bones, muscles, cartilage, skin, and blood. Carbohydrates are the primary energy source for the body, while fats store energy, insulate us and protect our vital organs. They each also affect our hormonal environment differently, which in turn influences our metabolism and weight.

In the context of a calorie-restricted diet like Dr. Now's, the precise balancing of these macronutrients becomes crucial not merely for maintaining daily functions but also for ensuring that you can lose weight without losing health. The ideal balance ensures that you can sustainably burn fat, minimize muscle loss, and maintain adequate energy levels.

To begin understanding this balance, one must first consider the individual roles of each macronutrient. Proteins are typically prioritized in weight loss diets due to their muscle-sparing properties and ability to induce satiety. Including sufficient protein in your diet helps safeguard your muscle mass, which is vital since muscle tissue burns more calories than fat tissue, even at rest. Carbohydrates, especially complex ones, are integral as they provide the energy required to fuel both brain function and physical activities. However, their consumption must be moderated and timed appropriately to avoid unnecessary insulin spikes that could lead to increased fat storage.

Fats, despite being high in calories, are essential for absorbing vitamins and providing essential fatty acids the body cannot produce on its own. The types of fats consumed can influence body weight and physiological functions. Thus, opting for sources of unsaturated fats can enhance your cardiovascular health and provide anti-inflammatory benefits.

Balancing these macronutrients means more than just hitting a daily calorie goal; it's about macronutrient distribution that aligns with one's metabolic health, physical activity level, and weight loss goals. Typically, a balanced distribution might look something like a plate divided into three parts: half of the plate filled with non-starchy vegetables (providing fiber and micronutrients with few carbs), one quarter with lean protein sources, and one quarter with healthy fat sources and/or whole grains.

For someone on a 1200-calorie diet, it might be useful to target specific ratios such as 40% of calories from carbohydrates, 30% from protein, and 30% from fats. However, these ratios can vary depending on individual factors including age, sex, physical activity level, and metabolic health. It's always advisable to adjust these ratios under professional guidance to tailor the diet to individual needs.

Moreover, the timing of macronutrient intake can also play a crucial role in balancing the diet effectively. For instance, consuming a higher proportion of carbohydrates in the morning could provide sufficient energy throughout the day, while tapering them off in the evening might help with utilizing fat stores for energy during sleep.

It's also vital to keep in mind that the quality of the macronutrients matters just as much as the quantity. Choosing whole, unprocessed foods can dramatically improve the quality of your diet. Whole foods are more nutrient-dense, supplying the vitamins and minerals that your body needs to function optimally.

This dietary balancing act is not just about shedding pounds; it's about crafting a sustainable way of living that promotes health. As you adjust your diet, consider each change as a step towards a deeper harmony between your body's needs and its goals. This isn't a temporary fix but a permanent transformation that requires mindful adjustments and an understanding of nutrition's complex, yet profoundly impactful role in your life.

CALCULATING YOUR MACROS

To begin, understanding your daily energy requirement is paramount. Everyone's body consumes a certain number of calories simply to maintain vital functions—at rest, our bodies burn calories to breathe, circulate blood, and regulate body temperature. This is known as Basal Metabolic Rate (BMR). The next layer includes physical activity. Even regular movements such as walking, typing, or cleaning add to your calorie needs. This total number, the sum of your BMR and calories burned through daily activities, outlines the energy your body requires each day.

From these calculations, setting up macronutrient targets involves accounting for what proportion of these calories should come from proteins, fats, and carbohydrates. Typically, a balanced approach for a weight loss regimen like the 1200-calorie diet might look like allocating 30% of your calories to proteins, 30% to fats, and 40% to carbohydrates. However, these proportions can shift depending on individual circumstances, preferences, or specific health goals.

Let's decipher what this translates to in the real world:

Step 1: Determining Your Caloric Needs

The first step is to calculate your BMR. Different formulas exist, but the Mifflin-St Jeor Equation is one of the most commonly used methods: - For men: BMR = 10 weight(kg) + 6.25 height(cm) - 5 age(y) + 5 - For women: BMR = 10 weight(kg) + 6.25 height(cm) - 5 age(y) - 161

From here, you adjust according to your activity level, multiplying your BMR by the factor that best describes your daily activity: - Sedentary (little or no exercise): BMR x 1.2 - Lightly active (light exercise/sports 1-3 days/week): BMR x 1.375 - Moderately active (moderate exercise/sports 3-5 days/week): BMR x 1.55 - Very active (hard exercise/sports 6-7 days a week): BMR x 1.725 - Super active (very hard exercise/physical job & exercise 2x/day): BMR x 1.9

Step 2: Setting Macronutrient Goals

Once you have an idea of your total calorie needs, dividing these calories by macronutrient percentages will give you a roadmap for your daily intake. For instance, if your calculation leads you to a need for 2000 calories per day, and you're following a 30% protein, 30% fat, and 40% carb plan: - Protein: 2000 x 0.30 = 600 calories from protein - Fat: 2000 x 0.30 = 600 calories from fat - Carbohydrates: 2000 x 0.40 = 800 calories from carbs

Next, convert these calorie values into grams, knowing that proteins and carbohydrates provide about 4 calories per gram, and fats provide about 9 calories per gram: - Protein: 600 / 4 = 150 grams of protein - Fat: 600 / 9 = ~67 grams of fat - Carbohydrates: 800 / 4 = 200 grams of carbs

Step 3: Applying This To Your Diet

Translating these macronutrient quantities into actual food can be an art form. It involves reading nutrition labels, measuring portions, and making educated food choices that align with these goals. Using tools such as digital food scales and apps can help track your intake precisely. However, it's also about quality—not all grams of carbohydrates or protein are created equal. Opting for whole, unprocessed foods can dramatically increase the nutrient density of your meals. Adjusting your macro ratios isn't strictly about rigid numbers; it's a fluid process that requires tuning into your body's reactions and adjusting based on progress and well-being. It's about finding the sweet spot where your body feels energized, your cravings are at bay, and your health metrics are moving in the right direction.

Macronutrient tracking and adjusting is essentially like being the conductor of an orchestra. Each section (protein, carbs, and fats) has a role to play, and when they come together harmoniously, they create a symphony of health and weight management that feels effortless and sustainable. Through calculated strategy and mindful eating, you orchestrate a dynamic balance that fuels your body's needs while fostering weight loss and well-being.

4. PORTION CONTROL AND SERVING SIZES

Imagine stepping into a quaint kitchen, where every ingredient has its place, and every serving size is a step towards your health goals. Portion control and serving sizes may sound rigid to some, but think of them as the subtle art of balance—a crucial element in your journey with the Dr. Nowzaradan's 1200-Calorie Diet.

In the tale of weight loss, portion control emerges not just as a chapter but as the narrative thread that binds the whole story together. The concept is deceptively simple: manage how much you eat and you can manage your weight. But as anyone embarking on this journey knows, simplicity often masks complexity.

Let's begin with a common scenario: you're at a dinner party, and a platter of grilled chicken is passed around. The tantalizing smell wafts towards you, your stomach grumbles, and before you know it, you've piled your plate high. It's only later, when tallying the day's calories, that the realization dawns—it was too much. Now, how does one navigate such a situation? By honing a skill that marries the eye with the mind: the visual estimation of portion sizes.

Visual guides are a cornerstone of portion control. It's much like learning to paint; at first, you follow the brushstrokes of the masters—measuring cups, scales, and guidelines help you understand the basics. Over time, though, you start to see nuances. A fist-sized serving of vegetables, a palm-sized portion of protein, a cupped hand of carbs. These images anchor your understanding, enabling you to 'eyeball' servings even when the tools aren't at hand.

Consider Sarah, a vibrant woman in her forties who found herself perplexed by portion sizes. Despite her best efforts, the scale seemed stuck. When she began using visual guides to control her portions, she realized she'd been serving herself twice the recommended amount of pasta at dinners. By adjusting her portions, she not only kickstarted her weight loss but also learned a valuable aspect of the diet: trust in one's own judgment.

Tools and techniques further refine this skill. Digital scales and measuring cups don't have to be your foes; they're the mentors that guide you towards autonomy. A small digital scale can be a revelation, showing you the true weight of a snack you might have underestimated. Over time, what once required checking and double-checking becomes second nature.

The story of portion control is never complete without a dialogue about adjusting portions to fit individual needs. Everyone's body responds differently to different diets. That's where understanding your personal basal metabolic rate (BMR) comes into play—knowing how much your body needs is the first step in feeding it correctly. This isn't just about reducing quantities; it's about aligning your intake with your body's actual energy requirements, which can fluctuate based on age, activity level, and even the climate you live in.

This chapter wouldn't be complete without addressing one of the most pervasive myths in dieting: that reducing portion sizes will leave you starving. Let me introduce you to Jack, who had always equated satisfaction with fullness to the brim. Jack learned that proper portion sizes often meant he finished his meal before feeling 'full', but within an hour, he realized he was indeed satisfied— without overeating. It's a subtle shift in mindset: from eating to absolute fullness, to eating for satisfaction and letting your body catch up.

Now, imagine that you, like Jack, have just started to master portion control. You sit down to dinner, and tonight's plate looks different. It's aligned with your newfound respect for portions— a bit more vegetables, a bit less starch. As you eat, you're aware, perhaps for the first time, of being in control—of knowing that this meal is just right for you. You're no longer eating passively; you are making decisions with every bite.

That sense of control—the empowering realization that you are in charge of your diet—is the true art behind portion control and understanding serving sizes. As you advance in your journey, remember that these are not constraints but tools designed to sculpt your pathway to a healthier life. They teach you moderation, awareness, and appreciation of food as not just sustenance but a cornerstone of your health.

THE IMPORTANCE OF PORTION CONTROL

In the realm of successful weight management, understanding and applying the art of portion control stands as a cornerstone, much like the keystone in an arch, providing both support and balance. For those engaging with Dr. Nowzaradan's 1200-Calorie Diet, grasping this concept is not just beneficial—it's essential.

Let us delve into the journey of Lisa, a committed dieter who learned that more isn't always merrier when it comes to food. Initially perplexed by her stalled weight loss, despite sticking religiously to her list of 'healthy' foods, Lisa's breakthrough came when she realized size does matter—in portions, that is.

At the heart of Lisa's story, and countless others', lies a simple truth: without portion control, even the healthiest of diets can falter. Consuming nutrient-rich, low-calorie foods can still lead to weight gain if eaten in large quantities. Herein lies the importance of portion control—it's not just about eating the right foods, but eating them in the right amounts.

Take, for instance, almonds. Rich in healthy fats, protein, and fiber, they're a powerhouse of nutrition. But a casual handful can easily turn into two or three, pushing calorie intake far beyond what one might assume. This is where the visual art of portion control comes into play.

Visualize this: A proper serving of almonds, roughly 23 nuts, fits snugly in the palm of your hand. In contrast, imagine an entire bag sitting on your desk as you work, tempting you to reach in repeatedly without thought. The difference in these scenarios isn't just in the amount consumed but in the mindfulness brought to eating. Portion control encourages us not just to eat, but to eat attentively, appreciating each bite and recognizing when we have had enough.

Portion control also harmonizes beautifully with calorie counting, a practice central to the Dr. Now Diet Plan. It empowers you to have a clear, quantitative understanding of what you consume, facilitating decisions that align with your weight loss goals. This synergistic relationship enables dieters to create a balanced, healthy eating pattern that fits within a daily caloric budget, making weight loss feel more like a manageable journey than a taxing quest.

Reflecting on the importance of portion control also brings us to the effect of oversized portions in our environment. Our plates have grown larger, our serving spoons longer, and our perception of 'normal' has shifted accordingly. This phenomenon isn't just a matter of personal choice; it's woven into the fabric of restaurant servings and packaged goods, making it a societal challenge as well.

Relearning how much to eat involves reprogramming these perceptions, a task that might seem daunting but is remarkably achievable with tools like smaller plates, cups, and bowls. These aren't just kitchen accessories; they're visual cues that guide your brain into accepting smaller servings as satisfying. The psychological influence of portion control cannot be overstressed. When you start seeing results from proper portioning, a positive feedback loop begins. Success breeds motivation, and motivation propels further success. This is evident in the story of Mark, who after two weeks of incorporating strict portion control, found his clothes looser and his energy levels heightened—tangible rewards that spurred him to steadfast commitment to his diet.

In addition to personal anecdotes, scientific studies bolster the argument for portion control's efficacy. Research indicates that people unknowingly consume more calories when presented with larger portions, a tendency that can be curbed by reducing plate size. Thus, the science not only supports the practice but also clarifies its mechanisms: by reducing visual cues associated with large quantities, we can trick our brains into feeling satisfied with less.

However, portion control does not mean perpetual restriction. It invites a deeper understanding of personal nutrition needs. Factors like age, gender, activity level, and metabolic health all play roles in determining the right portion sizes for an individual. Tailoring your portion control to fit these factors ensures that you're nourishing your body optimally without overfeeding it.

Moreover, integrating portion control doesn't require you to forgo your favorite foods. It's about balance. You can still enjoy a slice of pizza or a small dessert; it's the amount and frequency that matter. It's a liberating concept, really—knowing you don't have to eliminate foods but rather adjust how often and how much of them you consume.

VISUAL GUIDES FOR PORTION SIZES

Navigating the landscape of nutrition and dieting often takes you down a path lined with confusing measurements and ambiguous serving sizes. It's a common tale for many embarking on their weight loss journey, like Ellen, a teacher with a passion for healthy eating but a hectic schedule that made meticulous measuring a challenge. Her story and countless others underscore the profound utility of visual guides in mastering portion control—one of the most effective tools in ensuring dieting success.

Imagine walking into your kitchen, ready to prepare a meal under the guidelines of the 1200-Calorie Diet Plan. Instead of reaching for measuring cups and scales, you use a far simpler and readily available tool: your own hands. This method isn't just a clever trick—it's an empowering approach that enables quick and accurate portion sizing based on a few easy-to-remember visuals. Your hand, for instance, becomes more than just a part of your body; it's a bespoke measuring device tailored to your size and needs. A fist approximates a cup—ideal for gauging servings of vegetables or cooked pasta. Your palm, excluding fingers, offers a measure for the recommended three ounces of meat or fish, akin to a deck of cards. A cupped hand holds about half a cup—perfect for snacking on nuts or doling out a side of rice. Lastly, the tip of your thumb from knuckle to tip provides a tablespoon measure, particularly useful for gauging salad dressing or cream.

These visual approximations bring a practical elegance to dieting, allowing immediate judgment with minimal interruption to the cooking or eating process. Imagine Ellen's relief as she prepares her classroom snacks, swiftly assessing portions without pausing her ever-busy day. Such simplicity not only saves time but reinforces a sustainable habit of mindful eating.

However, the utility of visual guides extends beyond mere convenience. They play a crucial psychological role by clarifying and demystifying portion sizes, which can often be sources of misunderstanding in traditional numerical methods that suggest '30 grams' or 'a 100 calorie serving'. Instead, these visual cues provide tangible, understandable metrics that align closely with the eating experiences in everyday life.

Consider a dinner gathering, where the difference between feeling uncomfortably stuffed and perfectly satiated can lie in the seemingly simple decision of how much potato salad to spoon onto your plate. Here, visual guides act less like strict rules and more like friendly suggestions, whispered reminders that guide your choices towards moderation without dampening the joy of communal meals.

In addition to easing the individual's meal planning, visual guides also forge a deeper understanding and connection with food. When portions are measured with personal, intuitive tools like the hands and eyes, eating transforms from a quantified interaction to one that is qualitative and engaged. This sensory-based approach can lead to a more satisfying dietary experience where the eater becomes intuitively attuned to their body's needs and cues, fostering a harmonious eating behavior that diets often disrupt.

Beyond the individual kitchen or dining table, visual portion guides are equally pivotal in educational contexts, where they serve as universally accessible tools for teaching students and adults alike about healthy eating. They democratize nutritional knowledge, breaking down socioeconomic barriers that can complicate access to scale-based measuring tools.

This approach also warmly invites people back into the kitchen, an arena where modern convenience has often led to a reliance on pre-packaged, controlled portions, removing the eater further from the source of their sustenance. By using visual portion control methods, people re-engage with the process of cooking and serving food, reaffirming a hands-on connection that can be lost in today's fast-paced diet culture.

Visual guides for portion sizes stand out not just for their practicality and accessibility, but also for their ability to weave the act of eating back into the fabric of everyday life. They remind us that eating well isn't merely about following strict measurements or adhering rigidly to a diet. Instead, it's about developing an insightful, responsive relationship with food, where each meal becomes an opportunity to nourish both body and soul.

PORTION CONTROL TOOLS AND TECHNIQUES

In the narrative of achieving sustainable weight loss, portion control stands as a pivotal chapter. While the principles of portion control can feel abstract, the story becomes clearer and more actionable when we dive into the tools and techniques that bring this concept to life.

Take Michael, for example, a committed father and a busy lawyer, whose story is a familiar one of early morning rushes and late-night dinners. Like many, he knew the theory behind portion control but struggled in practice until he introduced specific tools and strategies into his daily routine. As Michael discovered, the integration of these tools not only streamlined his diet but also transformed his relationship with food from a source of stress to one of enjoyment and control.

Starting with one of the most fundamental tools—digital food scales—Michael learned to precisely measure his food. This kind of specificity, down to the gram, demystified calorie counting and helped him understand exactly how much he was consuming. This might seem meticulous, but it's akin to using a ruler instead of guessing the length of a piece of wood you need—if you want accurate results, precise tools are your best allies.

Beyond scales, measuring cups and spoons also became part of his arsenal. When preparing his morning oatmeal or serving out rice for dinner, these tools provided quick and effortless ways to keep his portions in check without always having to use a scale. Like bumpers in a bowling lane, they guided Michael's portions safely down the path of his calorie goals.

But technology has further refined the market of portion control. Consider smartphone apps, a tool that entered the stage of Michael's journey with great timing. Applications designed for tracking food intake and calories processed each entry, comparing it to his daily targets. This constant feedback loop—the immediate knowledge of 'budget' spent and remaining—proved invaluable in making real-time decisions about his meals.

Another effective technique comes not from gadgets or devices but from rethinking the dinnerware itself. By simply switching to smaller plates, Michael found that his servings visually filled the plate, satisfying his eyes as well as his stomach. This psychological trick, known as the less illusion, where people tend to fill plates regardless of their size, meant that smaller plates led to lesser food automatically, a subtle yet powerful tweak to his dining habit.

On that note, it's crucial to consider the layout of the environment. Michael, reaching another level in his journey, restructured his pantry and refrigerator. He placed healthier options at eye level and pre-portioned snacks into single-serving containers.

This not only made healthier choices easier but also added an extra step of consideration before he opted for less healthy indulgences lurking in the back.

Techniques matter as much as tools. One standout technique is the 'half-plate' rule, which Michael adopted during meals that were harder to measure, like family potlucks or buffet-style gatherings. By filling half his plate with vegetables and the rest with equal parts of proteins and carbohydrates, he managed to enjoy diverse foods while controlling portions and maintaining a balanced diet.

Creating and following these food rituals, Michael realized, was less about restriction and more about creating a structure within which he could enjoy food. This wasn't a diet in the traditional sense—it was a sustainable way of eating that allowed him to savor his meals without overindulging.

Moreover, the visual aspect of portion control reversibly educated his family, teaching them about balance and moderation in diet just by observation and participation. Michael's children, who saw their father use scales, measure portions, and choose smaller plates, imbibed these habits subconsciously, a ripple effect fostering a healthy environment at home.

In integrating these tools and techniques into your daily routine, remember, this transition to disciplined eating doesn't subtract from the joy of meals—it enhances it. You begin to appreciate quantities, quality, and the art of balance on your plate. Each meal becomes a testament to your control over your diet and, by extension, over your health trajectory.

As Michael's story unfolds, from battling diet misconceptions to mastering mindful eating, it serves as a motivating reminder that the right tools and a strategic approach can turn the challenge of portion control into a rewarding, life-changing habit. This proactive and equipped approach to dieting isn't just about losing weight—it's about gaining a lifestyle that celebrates food while respecting the body's needs.

SERVING SIZES FOR DIFFERENT FOODS

Picture the scene: a bustling holiday dinner where the table groans under the weight of varied, delicious foods. Here, understanding serving sizes for different foods is not merely a practice but a passport to enjoying this feast guilt-free. Learning about appropriate serving sizes is akin to mastering the language of your body's nutritional needs—it is a crucial skill for anyone looking to manage their weight effectively.

Sam's journey with portion sizes illustrates this beautifully. Like many, he struggled to maintain a balanced diet, especially given the rich diversity of foods available. His confusion wasn't rare— fruits, vegetables, proteins, and desserts each require different approaches when determining the right amount to eat. Only through truly understanding that each food group has unique serving size guidelines could Sam begin to navigate his diet more effectively. Take, for instance, proteins, foundational building blocks for our bodies. The ideal serving size can be visualized as roughly the size of a deck of cards. Consider the thickness and area when you look at a grilled chicken breast or a piece of salmon. This visualization provides a quick, reliable gauge for single servings at any meal and counters the common temptation to load up on extra protein, thinking it might be more beneficial.

Then, there are the carbohydrates, often demonized in the dieting world but essential to a balanced diet. A serving size for cooked grains, like rice or pasta, should resemble a rounded handful—approximately half a cup. This portion is satiating but not excessive, complimenting your meal rather than overwhelming it. For Sam, breaking down his need for visual and satisfying servings helped moderate his intake without feeling deprived.

Vegetables, those varied and vital components of any meal, allow for a bit more freedom. The typical serving size—a full cup for raw vegetables or half a cup for cooked—may almost seem overly generous. Yet, this reflects nutritional advice prioritizing vegetables due to their high nutrient density and low-calorie count, making them ideal for volume eating where you can enjoy more 'bulk' for fewer calories.

Take fruit serving sizes which also require attention. A small apple, a half-cup of chopped fruit, or roughly the size of a tennis ball provides a handy visual reminder. This portion control not only helps maintain caloric balance but also respects the fruit's natural sugar content, ensuring that even healthy sweets are consumed in healthy quantities.

However, fats, often the most misunderstood member of the dietary family, need precise judgment. A teaspoon of oil or a small pad of butter—about the size of a dice—is adequate for cooking purposes. Though seemingly minimal, these small quantities ensure that fat's calorie-dense nature doesn't lead to accidental overconsumption.

Sam learned that different foods not only require different portion sizes but also different considerations of their visual representations. His initial misunderstanding was no fault of his own; the subtleties of dietary balance can escape the best of us. As he began applying these visual approximations, his meals transformed. No longer a pile of this or a heap of that, each plate became a curated collection of nutritional adequacy.

Learning to visualize and practically apply different serving sizes for various food categories profoundly impacted his relationship with food. It wasn't about restriction but about appropriate consumption. He came to understand that his overindulgences were more a miscommunication between mind and plate than a failure of will. Embracing suitable serving sizes is like tuning an instrument—calibrating your meals not just for pleasure but for health and harmony with your body's needs. This calibration allows for a diet that is both satisfying and sustainable, recognizing that each food has its role and its proper place on the plate.

In integrating these principles into his daily life, Sam found a new confidence at family dinners and work lunches, and even the festive tables of the holiday season no longer seemed like navigational hazards. His is a testament to the powerful simplicity of understanding serving sizes—a story not of limitation, but of liberation and balance.

ADJUSTING PORTIONS FOR INDIVIDUAL NEEDS

Imagine being at a fresh market where every fruit, vegetable, and cut of meat is different in size, shape, and nutritional content. Just like these diverse offerings, every individual has unique dietary needs and objectives. As simple as it might seem to follow a universal guide to portion control, the truth is we must fine-tune our approach to fit our personal health mosaic. This narrative detailed right here explores the profound significance of tailoring portion sizes to individual needs, transforming generic dieting into a personalized nutrition strategy.

Meet Linda, a 42-year-old school teacher who decided to embark on a weight loss journey after several health scares. With a history of diabetes running in her family and her busy lifestyle making regular meals a challenge, Linda found the one-size-fits-all approach to portion control frustrating and demotivating. Her turning point came when she consulted a nutritionist who introduced her to the art of adjusting portion sizes based on personal health stats, activity levels, and even food preferences and tolerances.

Linda's case underscores that dietary needs are not just about managing weight but also about addressing specific health concerns. For instance, individuals with diabetes, like Linda, may need to manage carbohydrate intake more stringently, thereby requiring careful adjustments to the portions of grains and sugars compared to those without such considerations. This strategy doesn't skirt around the joys of eating but respects the body's unique biochemical responses to food.

The process of adjusting food portions starts with understanding one's Basal Metabolic Rate (BMR), which represents the number of calories needed to keep the body functioning at rest. This calculation considers age, gender, height, and weight, providing a calorie guideline. However, this number alone isn't enough. Activity level plays a crucial role—it amplifies the caloric needs and, by extension, the portion sizes of meals to fuel these activities.

For someone like Linda, who enjoys morning jogs, her caloric intake, particularly her complex carbohydrates and proteins, needed fine-tuning to ensure she was energized throughout the day. By adjusting her portions to include a slightly increased amount of whole grains in the morning, she found she could maintain her energy levels without compromising her weight loss goals.

Moreover, considerations for portion adjustments extend beyond metrics and measurements; they delve deep into the psychological relationship one has with food. Take the example of Jerry, a retiree with a significant amount of weight to lose, who had always found comfort in the size of his meals. Reducing his portion sizes too abruptly left him feeling unsatisfied and triggered overeating. By gradually reducing his portions and substituting part of his meals with high-volume, low-calorie foods like salads and soups, Jerry could manage his hunger and still enjoy the sensation of a full plate.

Individualized portion control also embraces the spectrum of life's stages. Pregnant women, for instance, have different nutritional requirements that might mean increased portions of certain foods like leafy greens for folate or fish for omega-3 fatty acids. Adolescents experiencing growth spurts might need increased caloric intake, reflecting their heightened energy needs. These adjustments ensure that at each life stage, the diet supports optimal health.

Then there's the element of cultural and ethical food choices influencing portion sizes. Vegetarians or vegans, like 30-year-old Emily, need to carefully plan their meals to include plant-based proteins in adequate portions to meet their protein requirements. This might mean larger servings of legumes, tofu, or quinoa compared to non-vegetarian diets where animal proteins are more concentrated.

In practical terms, adjusting portions for individual needs means equipping oneself with knowledge and tools. For Linda, a weekly planning session where she measured out and packed her grains, proteins, and vegetables was instrumental. This wasn't just meal prep; it was a strategic approach to personalizing her portion control, an integral part of her path to wellness.

Each story, be it Linda's, Jerry's, or Emily's, illustrates that portion control is not about stringent restrictions. Instead, it's about understanding and listening to your body's cues. It's about respecting each person's nutritional needs and replacing the 'diet' mindset with a 'nourishment' perspective.

5. COMMON MISCONCEPTIONS ABOUT WEIGHT LOSS

One of the most pervasive myths is the idea of the "starvation mode." Many fear that drastically lowering calorie intake can cause their metabolism to slow down to a crawl as the body clings onto every calorie to survive. However, while a prolonged severe calorie deficit may influence metabolic rates, the structured calorie reduction in a monitored plan like Dr. Now's is designed to promote weight loss without tipping the body into a genuine starvation response, which is much more extreme than most realize.

The human body is remarkably adaptable and does adjust its metabolic processes in response to calorie intake, but this adaptation is not as immediate or disabling as the myth suggests. Instead, when the body first experiences fewer calories, it starts to use stored fats for energy, which is exactly the goal of weight loss. Essentially, it's not about sending your body a signal of starvation, but rather a message to start utilizing its reserves more efficiently.

Equally misunderstood is the idea of weight fluctuations. Weight loss isn't a linear journey—day-to-day, even hour-to-hour, your body weight can change due to factors like fluid balance, food intake, and exercise. It's not uncommon to see a slight weight increase the day after a rigorous workout due to muscle inflammation and water retention. This is often where discouragement sets in, as many interpret these fluctuations as failures. Understanding that these are normal can help maintain motivation, and why we emphasize tracking progress over weeks and months, rather than days.

Then there are the carbohydrates. Oh, the poor, misunderstood carbohydrates. Carbs are often painted as the villain in weight loss stories. But they're crucial for energy, and when chosen wisely—think fiber-rich fruits, vegetables, and whole grains—they support rather than sabotage weight loss. The balance and type of macronutrients can indeed make a difference. In Dr. Nowzaradan's diet plan, it's not about eliminating carbs but understanding how to select them intelligently to maintain a satisfying diet while still adhering to a calorie limit.

Portion control is another area rife with myths. Yes, reducing portion sizes can help control calorie intake, but it's not just about eating less of everything. It's about understanding which foods can be consumed in larger volumes—like leafy greens, which are low in calories and high in nutrients—and which should be limited. That's where techniques and tools for portion control are not about restriction but about balance and understanding.

Finally, we must address the psychological aspect—our mindset. The belief that "I've tried and failed before, so why try again?" is a significant barrier. Each attempt at weight loss, regardless of its past success, teaches us something about our bodies and our needs. With every attempt, you gather more data about what works and what doesn't for your unique body chemistry and lifestyle. This doesn't mean a diet failed; it means you are one step closer to finding the formula that works for you.

As we clear the fog around these common misconceptions, we empower ourselves to approach weight loss with better tools and a clearer mindset.

DEBUNKING DIET MYTHS

Wading through the vast sea of dietary advice can feel like navigating a minefield of information and misinformation alike. It's no surprise that diet myths are prolific; they are often attractive because they promise dramatic results with minimal effort or understanding. Here, we take some of these myths head-on, unraveling them with the aid of science and practical wisdom.

One prevailing myth that often circulates in dieting communities is the notion that certain "miracle" foods can burn fat. The idea is compelling: eat this, and you'll slim down. However, no food can inherently burn fat. Foods that claim to have fat-burning properties, like grapefruit or green tea, can contribute to a healthy diet but will not magically dissolve fat. Weight loss occurs when there's a deficit between calories consumed and calories expended – a truth that is far less glamorous but essential for setting realistic expectations.

Another widespread belief is that eating late at night causes weight gain, regardless of what you consume. The underlying truth is more about total caloric intake over 24 hours than the specific timing of meals. If eating late at night pushes you over your calorie budget for the day, then yes, it might contribute to weight gain. But it's the excess calories, not the time of consumption, that is the culprit. This misunderstanding often leads people to impose unnecessary restrictions on themselves which can create a rebound overeating effect.

Similarly, the demonization of whole food groups, particularly carbohydrates, pervades the diet world. Low-carb diets are touted as the end-all solution for weight loss, and while reducing carbs might help some people reduce their overall calorie intake, it isn't a one-size-fits-all solution. Carbohydrates are a primary energy source for the body and play crucial roles, particularly for brain function and during physical activity. The key is to choose the right types of carbs — those that are high in fiber and low in added sugars and refined grains.

Furthermore, the "diet starts tomorrow" mentality deserves a mention here. This procrastination is grounded in the belief that dieting is an all-or-nothing approach. Such thinking not only postpones taking action but also sets the individual up for a cycle of guilt and bingeing. Successful weight management is a gradual, consistent journey, not a sudden dive into restriction followed by inevitable backsliding.

Then comes the myth of extreme dieting as the best way to lose weight. While aggressive calorie restriction will result in weight loss, it's not sustainable or healthy long-term. Such diets can lead to nutritional deficiencies, loss of muscle mass, and severe mental health strains. Instead, gradual changes that integrate into an individual's lifestyle are preferable and more sustainable over the long haul. It's also often assumed that if you're not seeing immediate results on the scale, your efforts are futile.

Weight loss is typically nonlinear, and there are many reasons why you might not see immediate changes on the scale. Water retention, muscle gain, and where you are in your digestive cycle play roles. Effective weight management measures progress in various ways, not just the number on the scale.

UNDERSTANDING WEIGHT FLUCTUATIONS

Imagine this: you've been following your diet strictly for a week, feeling good about your progress. You step onto the scale, and much to your dismay, the numbers have barely budged—or worse, they've gone up. This scenario is all too common and can be incredibly disheartening. However, weight fluctuations are a normal part of anyone's weight loss journey, and understanding this can significantly ease the mental burden that comes with the inevitable ups and downs.

Weight fluctuations are influenced by a variety of factors besides actual fat loss or gain. For instance, water retention can play a significant role. The body's water balance is affected by numerous factors including your dietary intake, such as salt and carbohydrates, which can cause the body to retain water. Also, hydration levels can fluctuate based on your environment, activities, and even hormonal changes. Women, for instance, may notice weight fluctuations during different phases of their menstrual cycle due to changes in hormone levels influencing water retention.

Another often overlooked factor is muscle gain. If you have been exercising, especially strength training, you might be gaining muscle while losing fat. Since muscle is denser and weighs more than fat, this can result in the scale staying the same or even increasing, even as you become healthier and your body composition improves. This is a positive development, as increased muscle mass boosts metabolism, aiding further weight loss and improving overall physical health. The digestive system itself also plays a role in body weight at any given moment. The weight of undigested food remains in the digestive tract until fully processed, which can add variability to the number you see on the scale. Moreover, variations in bowel movements or fluid intake can also see slight changes in your weight.

It's also critical to spotlight the psychological impact of watching the scale too closely. Fixating on daily weight can lead to unnecessary stress and can be misleading since it's influenced by so many variables unrelated to your progress. This emotional rollercoaster can affect your mental health and motivation, pushing you toward unhealthy behaviors in an attempt to see rapid changes. Instead of daily monitoring, consider weekly check-ins, which can provide a more accurate picture of your true weight loss trend over time.

Moreover, consider other means of measuring progress beyond the scale. Measuring inches lost, noting improvements in how your clothes fit, or tracking fitness progress, such as the ability to lift heavier weights or walk further without fatigue, can all offer encouragement and proof of your progress. These measures can often tell you more about your health and achievements than your weight alone.

Understanding that these fluctuations are normal and part of the process is key to maintaining your motivation and commitment to your health goals. Recognizing that weight isn't a perfect indicator of health allows you to maintain focus on what truly matters: developing healthy, sustainable habits and celebrating the many ways in which your body is becoming stronger, more capable, and healthier.

By shifting focus from the scale to internal signals like energy levels, mood improvements, and overall well-being, we can create a more forgiving and positive approach to weight loss and health. This holistic approach not only makes the journey more enjoyable but also ingrains the healthy habits that make long-term success more likely. Armed with this knowledge, the journey to weight loss becomes less daunting, more informed, and tuned to the natural rhythms and needs of your body, paving the way for true and lasting change.

THE TRUTH ABOUT "STARVATION MODE"

One of the most daunting myths that swirl around the world of dieting and weight loss is the fear-inducing phenomenon known as "starvation mode." It's a term that often pops up in conversations about dieting, especially when someone expresses worries about lowering calorie intake significantly. The concern is that by dropping calories too low, the body will somehow flick a survival switch, cling desperately to fat stores, and grind metabolism to a halt. This concept, though rooted in a kernel of physiological truths, is often blown out of proportion and misunderstood. Let's demystify this concept once and for all.

First, it's essential to understand where this idea comes from. Biologically speaking, your body is indeed designed to protect itself during times of starvation. When you significantly reduce calorie intake, your body, aiming to preserve life, does slow down its energy expenditure. This adaptive response evolved over millennia as a survival mechanism. In true starvation, the body will start to use muscle tissue for energy after depleting fat stores, which is the body's last-resort measure to keep vital organs functioning.

However, what many don't realize is that this drastic survival response—often referred to as "starvation mode"—does not kick in unless you are genuinely starving. It is not something that happens just because you skip breakfast or cut your calorie intake to a diet-prescribed 1200 calories per day. The diet levels designed in structured plans like Dr. Nowzaradan's are carefully calibrated to ensure they're low enough to yield weight loss yet sufficient to keep your body from any real risk of starvation. The confusion often lies in conflating the normal metabolic adaptations to dieting with the extreme, true starvation response. When you reduce calorie intake, your body adapts by slightly lowering its resting metabolic rate (RMR), a phenomenon known as adaptive thermogenesis. It's your body's way of becoming more fuel-efficient, similar to a car adjusting its fuel use during a long journey on limited gasoline. This adaptation can make weight loss more challenging over time but it's gradual and far from the dramatic plummet many fear.

In practical settings, when people claim that they've hit starvation mode, they're often experiencing a plateau in their weight loss journey. This plateau is usually due to the body adjusting to the calorie restriction, and possibly other factors like inconsistent dietary adherence or decreased initial water loss—not because the metabolism has stopped. It's a signal to reassess and adjust, not a verdict that your body is resisting weight loss.

Moreover, the key to successfully managing this metabolic adaptation lies in how you approach calorie reduction. A balanced diet that includes adequate protein and regular physical activity, particularly strength training, can help counteract the metabolic slowdown by sustaining lean muscle mass, which itself helps maintain a healthier metabolic rate.

Understanding and communicating these nuances is crucial because fearing starvation mode can lead people to avoid healthy, lower-calorie diets that would significantly benefit their health and weight loss goals. It can also lead to unhealthy cycles of overly restrictive diets followed by periods of binge eating, driven by the mistaken belief that they need to 'reset' their metabolism.

So, while it's wise to be mindful of not drastically under-eating, especially over long periods, the starvation mode myth should not deter you from following a sensible, structured diet plan. Diet plans, especially those like Dr. Nowzaradan's, are designed with a deep understanding of human physiology. They aim not to starve you but to create a manageable caloric deficit that leads to successful and sustainable weight loss. By demystifying and understanding what "starvation mode" truly is—and isn't—you are better equipped to approach your weight loss journey with confidence, guided by science rather than fear.

SEPARATING FACT FROM FICTION

In an era flush with information and competing perspectives, distinguishing legitimate nutritional science from well-marketed fiction is more challenging—and crucial—than ever. The health and wellness landscape is fraught with claims that can often lead earnest dieters astray. Empowered by understanding, however, we can navigate these waters and embrace dietary habits rooted in reality rather than folklore.

One of the most common stumbling blocks in understanding weight loss is the allure of quick fixes and silver bullets. Advertisements boasting instant results with minimal effort can be tempting. They tap into our inherent desire for immediate gratification. However, true health transformation doesn't come from a bottle or a fad diet; it comes from consistent, informed lifestyle changes. Weight loss supplements and diet pills often claim to provide an easy solution, but they can skew our understanding of what weight loss involves and occasionally pose risks due to unregulated formulations or side effects.

Additionally, the concept that dietary fat is an enemy of weight loss persists stubbornly in many circles despite decades of evolving nutrition science. The truth is, fats are essential. They help in hormone production, nutrient absorption, and provide a dense form of energy. The key is understanding the difference between saturated, trans fats, and healthier fats such as omega-3 and omega-6 fatty acids found in fish, nuts, and certain oils. Incorporating the right types of fat in moderation is essential for a balanced diet.

Another popular narrative is that cutting out gluten will lead to better health and quicker weight loss. For those with celiac disease or a genuine gluten intolerance, avoiding gluten is crucial. However, for the majority of people, gluten-containing foods are not inherently the issue; excess and processed foods are more problematic. Whole grains, which often contain gluten, are rich in nutrients and fiber and can be part of a perfectly healthy diet.

Technology also adds a layer of complexity to the web of weight loss information. Fitness trackers and apps can provide useful feedback on our physical activities and dietary habits, but they are not infallible. Devices that track calorie burn can overestimate or underestimate actual energy expenditure, and reliance on such technologies may obscure the foundational importance of listening to our bodies. Learning to understand and respond to your body's signals — hunger, fullness, and other cues — is crucial.

Moreover, the scale of personal testimony and anecdotal evidence has tremendous weight in the digital age, where personal blogs and social media amplify individual stories. While these stories can be inspiring and provide a personal touch to dietary advice, they often lack the scientific backing or fail to address the complexity of individual dietary needs.

It's crucial to base dietary choices on broader scientific research and verified studies rather than singular personal success stories, which might not be applicable to everyone.

The proliferation of diet "hacks" also suggests that there's always a simpler, previously undiscovered trick to losing weight. These can range from the timing of meals to "fat-burning" beverages. While nuances like meal timing can affect how we feel and perform during the day, they are unlikely to be the deciding factor in a successful weight loss journey. The foundational principles of good nutrition—balance, moderation, and consistency—are less sensational but significantly more effective.

Thus, separating fact from fiction in weight loss is not just about debunking myths but building a more informed understanding of what truly influences body composition and health. This requires a critical eye and the willingness to engage with scientific literature, to ask questions, and most importantly, to recognize that sometimes, the answers are less exciting than the questions. Long-lasting weight loss is a complex, multifaceted journey that integrates nutritional science, psychological well-being, and practical, sustainable habit changes.

HOW TO STAY INFORMED

Firstly, understanding the basics of nutritional science offers a solid foundation from which to assess new information. Basic knowledge about how your body processes food, the role of different nutrients, and what calories really are can transform your approach from following trends to understanding facts. This doesn't require a degree in nutritional science but a curiosity to understand fundamental concepts.

Choosing reputable sources for your information is paramount. In an age where everyone with a social media account can broadcast advice, it's essential to rely on information from experts who are continually involved in research and practice. These include registered dietitians, certified nutritionists, medical professionals, and respected institutions reputed for health research. Their insights are often vetted through rigorous peer review and are based on current, empirical data rather than anecdotal evidence.

Critical thinking is your ally. When you come across new dietary advice or a weight loss strategy, consider the source: Who is sharing this information? Are they qualified? Look also at the evidence: Is it supported by reputable scientific research? Beware of red flags like promises of quick fixes, dramatic results with little effort, or secrets that "doctors hate." Genuine health advice generally promotes gradual, sustainable practices and acknowledges that individual needs may vary. Staying updated with scientific literature may seem daunting, but it doesn't have to involve reading dense research papers. Many online platforms and journals now offer lay summaries or discuss the implications of new research in accessible formats. Subscribing to newsletters from trusted medical and health organizations or tuning into podcasts hosted by experts can also be an excellent way to stay informed about the latest research without getting overwhelmed by the scientific jargon.

Networking with professionals can further enhance your understanding and provide reliable channels of information. Building relationships with healthcare providers or joining community groups focused on health and nutrition can offer support and deepen your knowledge base. These relationships can be a source of motivation, accountability, and advice tailored to your personal health journey.

Moreover, learning to adopt a holistic perspective on health-related advice can be enlightening. Weight loss or management is not just about diet; it also encompasses factors like exercise, sleep, and mental health. An informed approach recognizes how these elements interact and affect your overall well-being. This integrative view helps in making decisions that are not just good for your waistline but for your whole body and mind.

Documenting your journey and the effects of different approaches can also provide personal insights that no generic advice can offer. Keep a journal or use an app to track what you eat, how you feel, and your physical health metrics over time. This data can help you understand what works best for your body, providing a personalized blueprint for your health decisions.

CHAPTER 3: BREAKFAST RECIPES

VEGGIE-PACKED BREAKFAST SCRAMBLE

PREPARATION TIME: 10 min

COOKING TIME: 10 min

MODE OF COOKING: Sautéing

SERVINGS: 2

INGREDIENTS:

- 4 large eggs
- 1/4 cup skim milk
- 1/2 cup diced bell peppers (red, green, yellow)
- 1/2 cup diced tomatoes
- 1/4 cup chopped spinach
- 1/4 cup diced onion
- 1 tsp olive oil
- Salt and pepper to taste

PROCEDURE:

1. In a bowl, whisk together eggs and milk until well combined.
2. Heat olive oil in a non-stick skillet over medium heat.
3. Add onion and bell peppers, sauté until softened (about 3-4 min).
4. Add tomatoes and spinach, cook for an additional 2 min.
5. Pour the egg mixture into the skillet and stir gently until the eggs are fully cooked.
6. Season with salt and pepper to taste before serving.

TIPS:

- Add a dash of hot sauce for a spicy kick.
- Serve with a side of whole grain toast.

NUTRITIONAL VALUES: Calories: 210, Fat: 14g, Carbs: 7g, Protein: 15g, Sugar: 3

GREEK YOGURT PARFAIT

PREPARATION TIME: 5 min

MODE OF COOKING: Assembling

SERVINGS: 1

INGREDIENTS:

- 1 cup non-fat Greek yogurt
- 1/2 cup mixed berries (blueberries, strawberries, raspberries)
- 2 Tbsp granola
- 1 tsp honey
- 1 Tbsp chopped nuts (optional)

PROCEDURE:

1. Spoon half of the Greek yogurt into a glass or bowl.
2. Add a layer of mixed berries and granola.
3. Top with the remaining Greek yogurt.
4. Drizzle honey on top and sprinkle with nuts if using.

TIPS:

- Use seasonal fruits for variety.
- Substitute honey with maple syrup if preferred.

NUTRITIONAL VALUES: Calories: 250, Fat: 6g, Carbs: 29g, Protein: 22g, Sugar: 18g

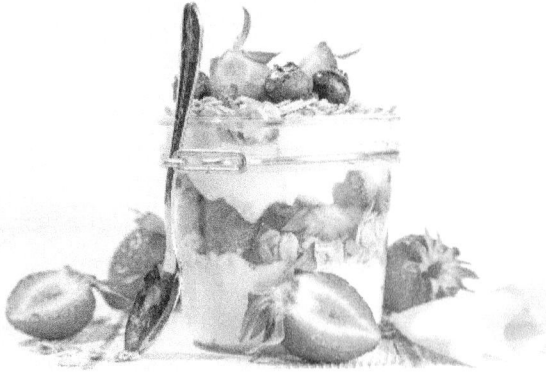

SPINACH AND FETA OMELETTE

PREPARATION TIME: 5 min

COOKING TIME: 10 min

MODE OF COOKING: Sautéing

SERVINGS: 1

INGREDIENTS:

- 2 large eggs
- 1/4 cup chopped spinach
- 2 Tbsp crumbled feta cheese
- 1 Tbsp skim milk
- 1 tsp olive oil
- Salt and pepper to taste

PROCEDURE:

1. In a bowl, whisk together eggs, milk, salt, and pepper.
2. Heat olive oil in a non-stick skillet over medium heat.
3. Add spinach and sauté until wilted (about 2 min).
4. Pour the egg mixture into the skillet and cook until the edges start to set.
5. Sprinkle feta cheese over the eggs.
6. Fold the omelette in half and cook until fully set.

TIPS:

- Serve with a side of fresh fruit for a balanced meal.
- Add diced tomatoes for extra flavor.

NUTRITIONAL VALUES: Calories: 200, Fat: 15g, Carbs: 2g, Protein: 14g, Sugar: 1g

BANANA OAT PANCAKES

PREPARATION TIME: 10 min

COOKING TIME: 15 min

MODE OF COOKING: Griddling

SERVINGS: 2

INGREDIENTS:

- 1 ripe banana
- 1/2 cup rolled oats
- 2 large eggs
- 1/2 tsp baking powder
- 1/2 tsp vanilla extract
- 1/4 tsp cinnamon
- Cooking spray

PROCEDURE:

1. In a blender, combine banana, oats,

eggs, baking powder, vanilla extract, and cinnamon.

2. Blend until smooth and let the batter sit for 5 min.

3. Heat a griddle or non-stick skillet over medium heat and coat with cooking spray.

4. Pour 1/4 cup of batter onto the griddle for each pancake.

5. Cook until bubbles form on the surface, then flip and cook until golden brown.

TIPS:

- Serve with fresh berries and a drizzle of honey.

- Add a tablespoon of Greek yogurt on top for extra protein.

NUTRITIONAL VALUES: Calories: 250, Fat: 8g, Carbs: 34g, Protein: 10g, Sugar: 8g

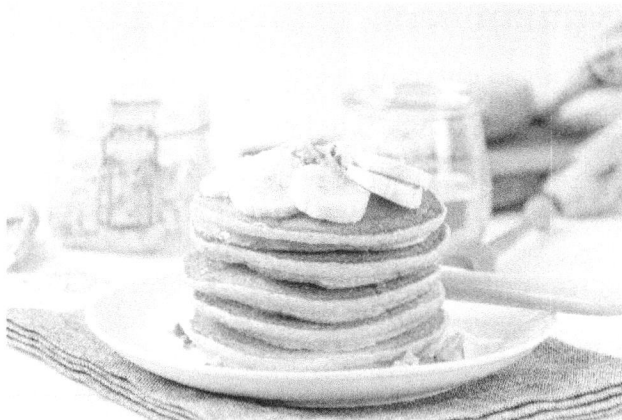

AVOCADO TOAST WITH POACHED EGG

PREPARATION TIME: 5 min

COOKING TIME: 5 min

MODE OF COOKING: Poaching

SERVINGS: 1

INGREDIENTS:

- 1 slice whole grain bread
- 1/2 ripe avocado
- 1 large egg
- 1 tsp lemon juice
- Salt and pepper to taste
- Red pepper flakes (optional)

PROCEDURE:

1. Toast the bread to your desired level of crispness.

2. In a small bowl, mash the avocado with lemon juice, salt, and pepper.

3. Spread the avocado mixture over the toasted bread.

4. Poach the egg in simmering water for 3-4 min until the white is set but the yolk remains runny.

5. Place the poached egg on top of the avocado toast and sprinkle with red pepper flakes if desired.

TIPS:

- Add sliced cherry tomatoes for a burst of freshness.

- Sprinkle with a little feta cheese for added flavor.

NUTRITIONAL VALUES: Calories: 220, Fat: 15g, Carbs: 18g, Protein: 9g, Sugar: 1g

CHIA SEED PUDDING

PREPARATION TIME: 5 min

COOKING TIME: 2 hr

MODE OF COOKING: Chilling

SERVINGS: 2

INGREDIENTS:

- 1/4 cup chia seeds
- 1 cup unsweetened almond milk
- 1 tsp honey
- 1/2 tsp vanilla extract
- Fresh fruit for topping

PROCEDURE:

1. In a bowl, combine chia seeds, almond milk, honey, and vanilla extract.
2. Stir well to mix and let sit for 5 min.
3. Stir again to prevent clumping, then cover and refrigerate for at least 2 hr or overnight.
4. Serve topped with fresh fruit.

TIPS:

- Mix in cocoa powder for a chocolate version.
- Top with nuts for added crunch.

NUTRITIONAL VALUES: Calories: 180, Fat: 9g, Carbs: 20g, Protein: 5g, Sugar: 6g

MIXED BERRY SMOOTHIE

PREPARATION TIME: 5 min

MODE OF COOKING: Blending

SERVINGS: 1

INGREDIENTS:

- 1/2 cup frozen mixed berries
- 1/2 banana
- 1 cup spinach leaves
- 1 cup unsweetened almond milk
- 1 Tbsp chia seeds

PROCEDURE:

1. Place all ingredients in a blender.
2. Blend until smooth.
3. Pour into a glass and enjoy immediately.

TIPS:

- Add a scoop of protein powder for an extra protein boost.
- Use coconut water instead of almond milk for a different flavor.

NUTRITIONAL VALUES: Calories: 160, Fat: 4g, Carbs: 28g, Protein: 4g, Sugar: 14g

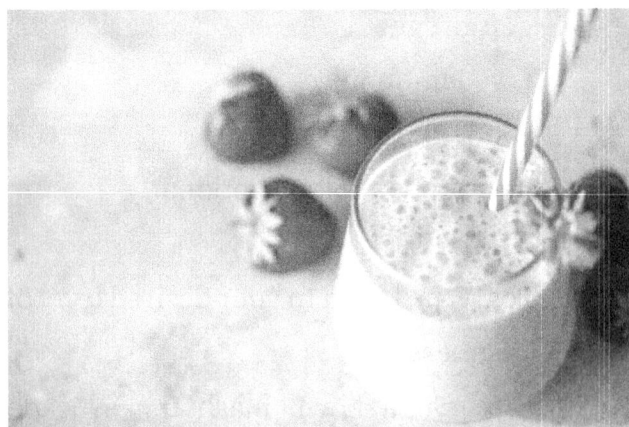

SWEET POTATO BREAKFAST BOWL

PREPARATION TIME: 10 min

COOKING TIME: 30 min

MODE OF COOKING: Baking

SERVINGS: 2

INGREDIENTS:

- 1 large sweet potato, peeled and diced
- 1 Tbsp olive oil
- 1/2 tsp cinnamon
- 1/4 tsp nutmeg
- 1 cup Greek yogurt
- 2 Tbsp honey
- 1/4 cup granola
- Fresh berries for topping

PROCEDURE:

1. Preheat oven to 400°F (204°C).
2. Toss diced sweet potatoes with olive oil, cinnamon, and nutmeg.
3. Spread on a baking sheet and bake for 25-30 min until tender.
4. In bowls, layer sweet potatoes, Greek yogurt, honey, granola, and fresh berries.

TIPS:

- Add a sprinkle of chia seeds for extra fiber.
- Drizzle with almond butter for additional flavor.

NUTRITIONAL VALUES: Calories: 300, Fat: 10g, Carbs: 45g, Protein: 10g, Sugar: 20g

COTTAGE CHEESE AND FRUIT BOWL

PREPARATION TIME: 5 min

MODE OF COOKING: Assembling

SERVINGS: 1

INGREDIENTS:

- 1 cup low-fat cottage cheese
- 1/2 cup pineapple chunks
- 1/4 cup blueberries
- 1 Tbsp chopped almonds
- 1 tsp honey

PROCEDURE:

1. Spoon cottage cheese into a bowl.
2. Top with pineapple chunks, blueberries, and almonds.
3. Drizzle honey over the top and serve.

TIPS:

- Substitute pineapple with any seasonal fruit.
- Sprinkle with a dash of cinnamon for extra flavor.

NUTRITIONAL VALUES: Calories: 220, Fat: 6g, Carbs: 24g, Protein: 20g, Sugar: 14g

APPLE CINNAMON OVERNIGHT OATS

PREPARATION TIME: 5 min

COOKING TIME: 6 hr

MODE OF COOKING: Chilling

SERVINGS: 1

INGREDIENTS:

- 1/2 cup rolled oats
- 1/2 cup unsweetened almond milk
- 1/4 cup unsweetened applesauce
- 1/2 tsp cinnamon
- 1/2 apple, diced
- 1 Tbsp chia seeds
- 1 tsp honey

PROCEDURE:

1. In a jar, combine oats, almond milk, applesauce, cinnamon, chia seeds, and honey.
2. Stir well to combine.
3. Add diced apple on top.
4. Cover and refrigerate overnight.
5. Stir before serving.

TIPS:

- Add a tablespoon of Greek yogurt for extra creaminess.
- Top with nuts or seeds for added texture.

NUTRITIONAL VALUES: Calories: 250, Fat: 7g, Carbs: 42g, Protein: 6g, Sugar: 12g

TOMATO AND BASIL EGG MUFFINS

PREPARATION TIME: 10 min

COOKING TIME: 20 min

MODE OF COOKING: Baking

SERVINGS: 4

INGREDIENTS:

- 6 large eggs
- 1/4 cup skim milk
- 1 cup cherry tomatoes, halved
- 1/4 cup chopped fresh basil
- 1/4 cup shredded mozzarella cheese
- Salt and pepper to taste
- Cooking spray

PROCEDURE:

1. Preheat oven to 375°F (190°C). Spray a muffin tin with cooking spray.
2. In a bowl, whisk together eggs, milk, salt, and pepper.
3. Evenly distribute cherry tomatoes and basil into the muffin tin cups.
4. Pour the egg mixture over the vegetables and top with shredded mozzarella.
5. Bake for 18-20 min, or until the egg muffins are set and golden brown.

TIPS:

- Store in the fridge for a quick breakfast option throughout the week.
- Add diced bell peppers or spinach for more veggies.

NUTRITIONAL VALUES: Calories: 110, Fat: 6g, Carbs: 2g, Protein: 10g, Sugar: 1g

QUINOA BREAKFAST BOWL

PREPARATION TIME: 5 min

COOKING TIME: 15 min

MODE OF COOKING: Boiling

SERVINGS: 2

INGREDIENTS:

- 1/2 cup quinoa
- 1 cup water
- 1/2 cup mixed berries
- 1/4 cup almond milk
- 1 Tbsp honey
- 1/4 tsp cinnamon
- 1 Tbsp chopped almonds

PROCEDURE:

1. Rinse quinoa under cold water.
2. In a saucepan, bring water to a boil. Add quinoa, reduce heat, and simmer for 15 min or until water is absorbed.
3. Stir in almond milk, honey, and cinnamon.
4. Divide quinoa into bowls, top with mixed berries and almonds.

TIPS:

- Prepare quinoa the night before for a quick breakfast.
- Substitute almond milk with your preferred milk.

NUTRITIONAL VALUES: Calories: 220, Fat: 5g, Carbs: 38g, Protein: 6g, Sugar: 12g

SMOKED SALMON AND AVOCADO TOAST

PREPARATION TIME: 5 min

COOKING TIME: 5 min

MODE OF COOKING: Assembling

SERVINGS: 1

INGREDIENTS:

- 1 slice whole grain bread
- 1/2 ripe avocado
- 2 oz smoked salmon
- 1 tsp lemon juice
- Salt and pepper to taste
- Fresh dill (optional)

PROCEDURE:

1. Toast the whole grain bread.
2. Mash avocado with lemon juice, salt, and pepper.
3. Spread the avocado mixture on the toasted bread.
4. Top with smoked salmon and garnish with fresh dill if desired.

TIPS:

- Add a poached egg on top for extra protein.
- Use multi-grain crackers for a lower-calorie option.

NUTRITIONAL VALUES: Calories: 250, Fat: 15g, Carbs: 20g, Protein: 13g, Sugar: 1g

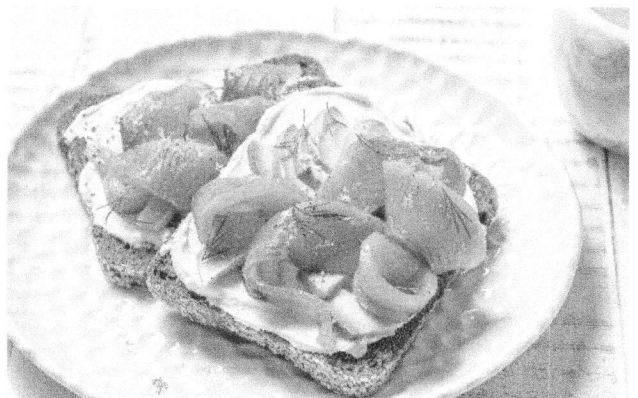

PROTEIN-PACKED SMOOTHIE BOWL

PREPARATION TIME: 5 min

MODE OF COOKING: Blending

SERVINGS: 1

INGREDIENTS:

- 1 frozen banana
- 1/2 cup frozen mixed berries
- 1/2 cup Greek yogurt
- 1/4 cup unsweetened almond milk
- 1 Tbsp chia seeds
- 1 scoop protein powder
- Fresh fruit and granola for topping

PROCEDURE:

1. Blend frozen banana, mixed berries, Greek yogurt, almond milk, chia seeds, and protein powder until smooth.
2. Pour into a bowl and top with fresh fruit and granola.

TIPS:

- Use coconut water instead of almond milk for a different flavor.
- Add a handful of spinach for extra nutrients.

NUTRITIONAL VALUES: Calories: 300, Fat: 6g, Carbs: 45g, Protein: 20g, Sugar: 20g

SAVORY OATMEAL WITH SPINACH AND EGG

PREPARATION TIME: 5 min

COOKING TIME: 10 min

MODE OF COOKING: Boiling and Sautéing

SERVINGS: 1

INGREDIENTS:

- 1/2 cup rolled oats
- 1 cup water
- 1 cup fresh spinach
- 1 large egg
- 1 tsp olive oil
- Salt and pepper to taste
- 1 Tbsp grated Parmesan cheese

PROCEDURE:

1. In a saucepan, bring water to a boil and add oats. Cook according to package instructions.
2. In a skillet, heat olive oil over medium heat. Sauté spinach until wilted.
3. Cook the egg sunny-side up or to your preference.
4. Combine cooked oats and spinach in a bowl. Top with the egg and sprinkle with Parmesan cheese, salt, and pepper.

TIPS:

- Add a splash of hot sauce for extra flavor.
- Use kale instead of spinach for a different twist.

NUTRITIONAL VALUES: Calories: 280, Fat: 12g, Carbs: 32g, Protein: 14g, Sugar: 1g

BLUEBERRY ALMOND OVERNIGHT OATS

PREPARATION TIME: 5 min

COOKING TIME: 6 hr

MODE OF COOKING: Chilling

SERVINGS: 1

INGREDIENTS:

- 1/2 cup rolled oats
- 1/2 cup unsweetened almond milk
- 1/4 cup fresh blueberries
- 1 Tbsp almond butter
- 1 Tbsp chia seeds
- 1 tsp honey

PROCEDURE:

1. In a jar, combine oats, almond milk, blueberries, almond butter, chia seeds, and honey.
2. Stir well to combine.
3. Cover and refrigerate overnight.
4. Stir before serving.

TIPS:

- Add a sprinkle of cinnamon for extra flavor.
- Use frozen blueberries if fresh are not available.

NUTRITIONAL VALUES: Calories: 290, Fat: 12g, Carbs: 40g, Protein: 8g, Sugar: 10g

COTTAGE CHEESE AND VEGGIE BOWL

PREPARATION TIME: 5 min

MODE OF COOKING: Assembling

SERVINGS: 1

INGREDIENTS:

- 1 cup low-fat cottage cheese
- 1/2 cup cherry tomatoes, halved
- 1/4 cup diced cucumber
- 1/4 cup diced bell peppers
- 1 Tbsp chopped fresh parsley
- Salt and pepper to taste

PROCEDURE:

1. Spoon cottage cheese into a bowl.
2. Top with cherry tomatoes, cucumber, bell peppers, and parsley.
3. Season with salt and pepper and serve.

TIPS:

- Add a drizzle of balsamic glaze for extra flavor.
- Serve with whole grain crackers for added texture.

NUTRITIONAL VALUES: Calories: 200, Fat: 4g, Carbs: 16g, Protein: 28g, Sugar: 6g

PEANUT BUTTER BANANA SMOOTHIE

PREPARATION TIME: 5 min

MODE OF COOKING: Blending

SERVINGS: 1

INGREDIENTS:

- 1 ripe banana
- 1 cup unsweetened almond milk
- 1 Tbsp natural peanut butter
- 1/2 tsp vanilla extract
- 1 scoop protein powder (optional)
- Ice cubes

PROCEDURE:

1. Place all ingredients in a blender.
2. Blend until smooth.
3. Pour into a glass and enjoy immediately.

TIPS:

- Use frozen banana for a thicker smoothie.
- Add a handful of spinach for extra nutrients.

NUTRITIONAL VALUES: Calories: 250, Fat: 8g, Carbs: 35g, Protein: 10g, Sugar: 18g

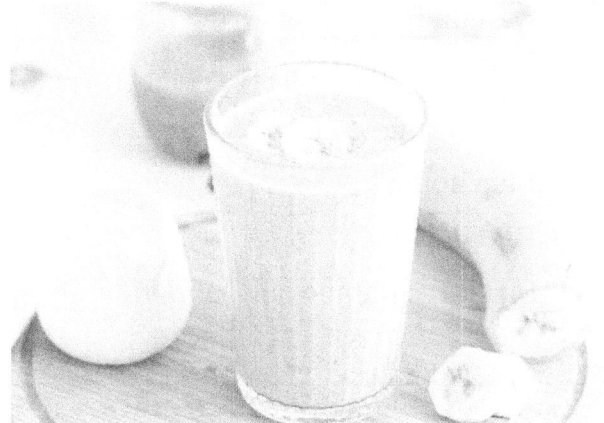

BROCCOLI AND CHEESE BREAKFAST BURRITO

PREPARATION TIME: 10 min

COOKING TIME: 10 min

MODE OF COOKING: Sautéing

SERVINGS: 2

INGREDIENTS:

- 4 large eggs
- 1/4 cup skim milk
- 1 cup chopped broccoli
- 1/4 cup shredded cheddar cheese
- 1 tsp olive oil
- Salt and pepper to taste
- 2 whole wheat tortillas

PROCEDURE:

1. In a bowl, whisk together eggs, milk, salt, and pepper.
2. Heat olive oil in a non-stick skillet over medium heat.
3. Add broccoli and sauté until tender.
4. Pour egg mixture into the skillet and cook until eggs are scrambled and fully cooked.
5. Divide the egg and broccoli mixture between the tortillas and top with shredded cheese.
6. Roll up the tortillas and serve.

TIPS:

- Add salsa for extra flavor.
- Substitute broccoli with spinach or kale.

NUTRITIONAL VALUES: Calories: 320, Fat: 14g, Carbs: 28g, Protein: 18g, Sugar: 2g

---

BAKED APPLE WITH CINNAMON AND WALNUTS

PREPARATION TIME: 10 min

COOKING TIME: 30 min

MODE OF COOKING: Baking

SERVINGS: 2

INGREDIENTS:

- 2 large apples, cored
- 2 tsp cinnamon
- 2 Tbsp chopped walnuts
- 2 tsp honey
- 1/2 cup Greek yogurt (optional)

PROCEDURE:

1. Preheat oven to 350°F (175°C).
2. Place apples in a baking dish.
3. Sprinkle cinnamon inside each apple and fill with chopped walnuts.
4. Drizzle honey over the top.
5. Bake for 30 min or until apples are tender.
6. Serve warm with a dollop of Greek yogurt if desired.

TIPS:

- Use pecans instead of walnuts for a different flavor.
- Add a sprinkle of nutmeg for extra spice.

NUTRITIONAL VALUES: Calories: 200, Fat: 8g, Carbs: 34g, Protein: 2g, Sugar: 24g

CHAPTER 4: LUNCH RECIPES

GRILLED CHICKEN SALAD WITH HONEY MUSTARD DRESSING

PREPARATION TIME: 15 min

COOKING TIME: 15 min

MODE OF COOKING: Grilling

SERVINGS: 2

INGREDIENTS:

- 2 boneless, skinless chicken breasts
- 4 cups mixed greens (lettuce, spinach, arugula)
- 1/2 cup cherry tomatoes, halved
- 1/4 cup sliced cucumber
- 1/4 cup shredded carrots
- 1/4 cup red onion, thinly sliced
- 2 Tbsp honey
- 1 Tbsp Dijon mustard
- 2 Tbsp olive oil
- 1 Tbsp apple cider vinegar
- Salt and pepper to taste

PROCEDURE:

1. Preheat grill to medium-high heat.
2. Season chicken breasts with salt and pepper.
3. Grill chicken for 6-7 min per side, or until fully cooked.
4. Let the chicken rest for 5 min, then slice.
5. In a small bowl, whisk together honey, Dijon mustard, olive oil, and apple cider vinegar to make the dressing.
6. In a large bowl, combine mixed greens, cherry tomatoes, cucumber, carrots, and red onion.
7. Top salad with sliced chicken and drizzle with honey mustard dressing.

TIPS:

- Add avocado slices for extra creaminess.
- Substitute grilled shrimp for chicken for variety.

NUTRITIONAL VALUES: Calories: 320, Fat: 14g, Carbs: 22g, Protein: 28g, Sugar: 14g

QUINOA AND BLACK BEAN STUFFED PEPPERS

PREPARATION TIME: 15 min

COOKING TIME: 30 min

MODE OF COOKING: Baking

SERVINGS: 4

INGREDIENTS:

- 4 large bell peppers, tops cut off and seeds removed
- 1 cup cooked quinoa
- 1 can (15 oz) black beans, drained and rinsed
- 1 cup corn kernels
- 1 cup diced tomatoes
- 1/2 cup diced onion
- 1/2 cup shredded cheddar cheese
- 1 tsp cumin
- 1 tsp chili powder
- Salt and pepper to taste

PROCEDURE:

1. Preheat oven to 375°F (190°C).
2. In a large bowl, combine quinoa, black beans, corn, tomatoes, onion, cumin, chili powder, salt, and pepper.
3. Stuff the bell peppers with the quinoa mixture.
4. Place stuffed peppers in a baking dish and top with shredded cheese.
5. Bake for 30 min or until the peppers are tender and the cheese is melted.

TIPS:

- Use different colored bell peppers for a vibrant presentation.
- Serve with a side of guacamole for added flavor.

NUTRITIONAL VALUES: Calories: 280, Fat: 8g, Carbs: 40g, Protein: 12g, Sugar: 6g

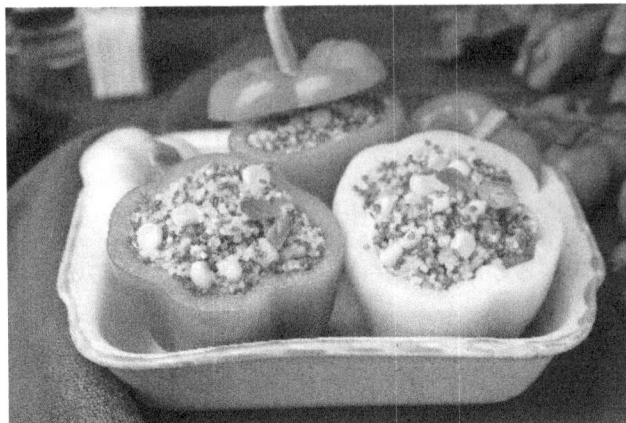

TURKEY AND AVOCADO WRAP

PREPARATION TIME: 10 min

MODE OF COOKING: Assembling

SERVINGS: 2

INGREDIENTS:

- 4 whole wheat tortillas
- 8 oz sliced turkey breast
- 1 ripe avocado, sliced
- 1/2 cup shredded lettuce
- 1/2 cup diced tomatoes
- 1/4 cup shredded cheese
- 2 Tbsp Greek yogurt
- 1 Tbsp Dijon mustard

PROCEDURE:

1. In a small bowl, mix Greek yogurt and Dijon mustard.
2. Lay out tortillas and spread the yogurt-mustard mixture evenly on each.
3. Layer turkey slices, avocado, lettuce, tomatoes, and cheese on each tortilla.
4. Roll up the tortillas tightly and cut in half before serving.

TIPS:

- Add a splash of hot sauce for extra spice.
- Substitute the turkey with grilled chicken or roast beef.

NUTRITIONAL VALUES: Calories: 350, Fat: 18g, Carbs: 30g, Protein: 22g, Sugar: 3g

LENTIL AND VEGGIE STIR-FRY

PREPARATION TIME: 10 min

COOKING TIME: 20 min

MODE OF COOKING: Sautéing

SERVINGS: 4

INGREDIENTS:

- 1 cup dried lentils
- 2 cups vegetable broth
- 1 cup broccoli florets
- 1 cup sliced bell peppers
- 1 cup sliced carrots
- 1/2 cup sliced onions
- 2 cloves garlic, minced
- 1 Tbsp olive oil
- 2 Tbsp soy sauce
- 1 Tbsp sesame oil
- 1 tsp grated ginger
- Salt and pepper to taste

PROCEDURE:

1. Rinse lentils and cook in vegetable broth according to package instructions.
2. In a large skillet, heat olive oil over medium heat. Add garlic and ginger, sauté until fragrant.
3. Add onions, carrots, broccoli, and bell peppers. Cook until vegetables are tender.
4. Stir in cooked lentils, soy sauce, and sesame oil. Cook for an additional 5 min.
5. Season with salt and pepper to taste before serving.

TIPS:

- Top with chopped green onions and sesame seeds.
- Serve over brown rice or quinoa for a complete meal.

NUTRITIONAL VALUES: Calories: 320, Fat: 10g, Carbs: 45g, Protein: 12g, Sugar: 6g

GREEK CHICKPEA SALAD

PREPARATION TIME: 10 min

MODE OF COOKING: Assembling

SERVINGS: 4

INGREDIENTS:

- 1 can (15 oz) chickpeas, drained and rinsed
- 1 cup cherry tomatoes, halved
- 1/2 cup diced cucumber
- 1/4 cup red onion, thinly sliced
- 1/4 cup Kalamata olives, pitted and sliced
- 1/4 cup crumbled feta cheese
- 2 Tbsp olive oil
- 1 Tbsp red wine vinegar
- 1 tsp dried oregano
- Salt and pepper to taste

PROCEDURE:

1. In a large bowl, combine chickpeas, cherry tomatoes, cucumber, red onion, olives, and feta cheese.

2. In a small bowl, whisk together olive oil, red wine vinegar, oregano, salt, and pepper.

3. Pour dressing over the salad and toss to combine.

TIPS:

- Add chopped fresh herbs like parsley or mint for extra freshness.
- Serve with whole grain pita bread.

NUTRITIONAL VALUES: Calories: 280, Fat: 14g, Carbs: 30g, Protein: 8g, Sugar: 3g

---

SPINACH AND MUSHROOM QUESADILLA

PREPARATION TIME: 10 min

COOKING TIME: 10 min

MODE OF COOKING: Sautéing and Griddling

SERVINGS: 2

INGREDIENTS:

- 4 whole wheat tortillas
- 1 cup fresh spinach
- 1/2 cup sliced mushrooms
- 1/2 cup shredded mozzarella cheese
- 1/4 cup diced onions
- 1 Tbsp olive oil
- Salt and pepper to taste

PROCEDURE:

1. Heat olive oil in a skillet over medium heat. Add onions and mushrooms, sauté until tender.

2. Add spinach and cook until wilted. Season with salt and pepper.

3. Place tortillas on a griddle or large skillet over medium heat.

4. Spread the vegetable mixture evenly over two tortillas and sprinkle with cheese.

5. Top with the remaining tortillas and cook until golden brown on both sides and cheese is melted.

6. Cut into wedges and serve.

TIPS:

- Add a side of salsa or Greek yogurt for dipping.
- Include bell peppers for extra flavor and nutrients.

NUTRITIONAL VALUES: Calories: 300, Fat: 14g, Carbs: 28g, Protein: 14g, Sugar: 3g

---

TURKEY MEATBALL AND VEGGIE SOUP

PREPARATION TIME: 15 min

COOKING TIME: 30 min

MODE OF COOKING: Boiling

SERVINGS: 4

INGREDIENTS:

- 1 lb ground turkey
- 1/4 cup breadcrumbs
- 1 egg
- 1 tsp garlic powder
- 1 tsp onion powder
- 1 tsp Italian seasoning
- Salt and pepper to taste

- 6 cups low-sodium chicken broth
- 1 cup diced carrots
- 1 cup diced celery
- 1 cup diced zucchini
- 1/2 cup diced onions
- 2 cups fresh spinach

PROCEDURE:

1. In a bowl, combine ground turkey, breadcrumbs, egg, garlic powder, onion powder, Italian seasoning, salt, and pepper. Form into small meatballs.
2. In a large pot, bring chicken broth to a boil. Add meatballs and cook for 10 min.
3. Add carrots, celery, zucchini, and onions. Simmer for 15 min or until vegetables are tender.
4. Stir in fresh spinach and cook until wilted. Season with salt and pepper before serving.

TIPS:

- Serve with a slice of whole grain bread.
- Add a splash of lemon juice for a fresh finish.

NUTRITIONAL VALUES: Calories: 250, Fat: 10g, Carbs: 20g, Protein: 22g, Sugar: 4g

---

CHICKEN AND VEGGIE STIR-FRY

PREPARATION TIME: 10 min

COOKING TIME: 15 min

MODE OF COOKING: Sautéing

SERVINGS: 4

INGREDIENTS:

- 2 boneless, skinless chicken breasts, sliced thinly
- 1 cup broccoli florets
- 1 cup sliced bell peppers
- 1 cup snap peas
- 1/2 cup sliced carrots
- 2 cloves garlic, minced
- 1 Tbsp olive oil
- 2 Tbsp soy sauce
- 1 Tbsp honey
- 1 tsp sesame oil
- Salt and pepper to taste

PROCEDURE:

1. In a large skillet, heat olive oil over medium-high heat. Add chicken and cook until browned.
2. Add garlic and cook until fragrant.
3. Add broccoli, bell peppers, snap peas, and carrots. Sauté until vegetables are tender.
4. Stir in soy sauce, honey, and sesame oil. Cook for another 2 min.
5. Season with salt and pepper before serving.

TIPS:

- Serve over brown rice or quinoa.
- Add red pepper flakes for a spicy kick.

NUTRITIONAL VALUES: Calories: 300, Fat: 12g, Carbs: 20g, Protein: 28g, Sugar: 7g

SALMON AND AVOCADO SALAD

PREPARATION TIME: 10 min

COOKING TIME: 15 min

MODE OF COOKING: Grilling

SERVINGS: 2

INGREDIENTS:

- 2 salmon fillets
- 4 cups mixed greens
- 1 ripe avocado, sliced
- 1/2 cup cherry tomatoes, halved
- 1/4 cup sliced cucumber
- 2 Tbsp olive oil
- 1 Tbsp lemon juice
- 1 tsp Dijon mustard
- Salt and pepper to taste

PROCEDURE:

1. Preheat grill to medium-high heat.
2. Season salmon fillets with salt and pepper.
3. Grill salmon for 6-8 min per side, or until fully cooked.
4. In a small bowl, whisk together olive oil, lemon juice, Dijon mustard, salt, and pepper to make the dressing.
5. In a large bowl, combine mixed greens, avocado, cherry tomatoes, and cucumber.
6. Top salad with grilled salmon and drizzle with dressing.

TIPS:

- Add hard-boiled eggs for extra protein.
- Substitute grilled chicken for salmon if preferred.

NUTRITIONAL VALUES: Calories: 350, Fat: 20g, Carbs: 15g, Protein: 30g, Sugar: 3g

VEGETARIAN SUSHI ROLLS

PREPARATION TIME: 20 min

COOKING TIME: 10 min

MODE OF COOKING: Rolling

SERVINGS: 2

INGREDIENTS:

- 1 cup sushi rice
- 1 1/2 cups water
- 2 Tbsp rice vinegar
- 1/2 tsp salt
- 1/2 tsp sugar
- 4 nori sheets
- 1/2 cucumber, julienned
- 1/2 avocado, sliced
- 1/2 carrot, julienned
- 1/2 bell pepper, julienned
- Soy sauce for serving

PROCEDURE:

1. Rinse sushi rice under cold water until water runs clear.
2. Combine rice and water in a saucepan, bring to a boil. Reduce heat, cover, and simmer for 10 min.
3. Remove from heat and let stand, covered, for 10 min.
4. In a small bowl, mix rice vinegar, salt, and sugar. Stir into cooked rice.

5. Place a nori sheet on a bamboo sushi mat, shiny side down. Spread an even layer of rice over nori, leaving a 1-inch border at the top.

6. Arrange cucumber, avocado, carrot, and bell pepper in a line across the center of the rice.

7. Roll up tightly using the bamboo mat, then slice into pieces.

TIPS:

- Serve with pickled ginger and wasabi.
- Use different vegetables for variety.

NUTRITIONAL VALUES: Calories: 250, Fat: 7g, Carbs: 40g, Protein: 4g, Sugar: 3g

---

CHICKEN CAESAR SALAD WRAP

PREPARATION TIME: 10 min

COOKING TIME: 10 min

MODE OF COOKING: Assembling

SERVINGS: 2

INGREDIENTS:

- 2 whole wheat tortillas
- 2 grilled chicken breasts, sliced
- 2 cups chopped romaine lettuce
- 1/4 cup grated Parmesan cheese
- 1/4 cup Caesar dressing
- 1/4 cup croutons (optional)

PROCEDURE:

1. Lay out tortillas on a flat surface.

2. In a bowl, combine chicken, lettuce, Parmesan cheese, and Caesar dressing.

3. Divide the mixture evenly between the two tortillas.

4. Roll up the tortillas tightly and cut in half before serving.

TIPS:

- Add cherry tomatoes for extra flavor.
- Use low-fat Caesar dressing to reduce calories.

NUTRITIONAL VALUES: Calories: 350, Fat: 14g, Carbs: 28g, Protein: 25g, Sugar: 3g

---

MEDITERRANEAN QUINOA SALAD

PREPARATION TIME: 15 min

COOKING TIME: 15 min

MODE OF COOKING: Boiling

SERVINGS: 4

INGREDIENTS:

- 1 cup quinoa
- 2 cups water
- 1/2 cup diced cucumber
- 1/2 cup diced tomatoes
- 1/4 cup diced red onion
- 1/4 cup Kalamata olives, sliced
- 1/4 cup crumbled feta cheese
- 2 Tbsp olive oil
- 1 Tbsp lemon juice
- 1 tsp dried oregano
- Salt and pepper to taste

PROCEDURE:

1. Rinse quinoa under cold water.

2. In a saucepan, bring water to a boil. Add quinoa, reduce heat, and simmer

for 15 min or until water is absorbed.

3. Let quinoa cool slightly.

4. In a large bowl, combine quinoa, cucumber, tomatoes, red onion, olives, and feta cheese.

5. In a small bowl, whisk together olive oil, lemon juice, oregano, salt, and pepper.

6. Pour dressing over the salad and toss to combine.

TIPS:

- Add grilled chicken for extra protein.

- Serve chilled for a refreshing meal.

NUTRITIONAL VALUES: Calories: 280, Fat: 12g, Carbs: 34g, Protein: 8g, Sugar: 3g

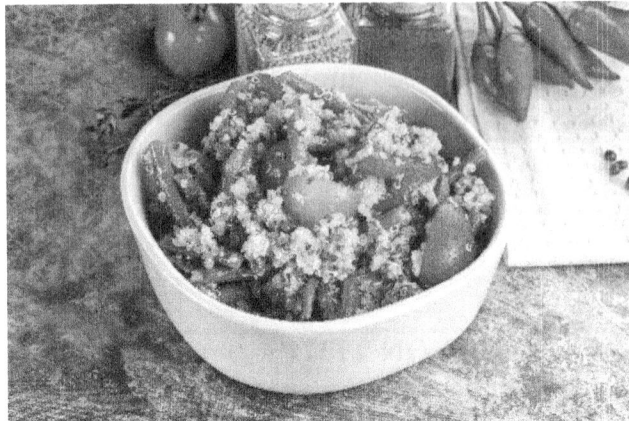

SHRIMP AND AVOCADO SALAD

PREPARATION TIME: 10 min

COOKING TIME: 5 min

MODE OF COOKING: Sautéing

SERVINGS: 2

INGREDIENTS:

- 1/2 lb shrimp, peeled and deveined
- 1 avocado, diced
- 2 cups mixed greens
- 1/2 cup cherry tomatoes, halved
- 1/4 cup red onion, thinly sliced
- 1 Tbsp olive oil
- 1 Tbsp lemon juice
- Salt and pepper to taste

PROCEDURE:

1. Heat olive oil in a skillet over medium heat.

2. Add shrimp and cook until pink and opaque, about 3-4 min per side.

3. In a large bowl, combine mixed greens, avocado, cherry tomatoes, and red onion.

4. Add cooked shrimp to the salad.

5. Drizzle with lemon juice, season with salt and pepper, and toss to combine.

TIPS:

- Add a sprinkle of feta cheese for extra flavor.
- Serve with a whole grain roll.

NUTRITIONAL VALUES: Calories: 300, Fat: 18g, Carbs: 12g, Protein: 24g, Sugar: 2g

SWEET POTATO AND BLACK BEAN TACOS

PREPARATION TIME: 10 min

COOKING TIME: 20 min

MODE OF COOKING: Baking

SERVINGS: 4

INGREDIENTS:

- 2 medium sweet potatoes, peeled and diced
- 1 can (15 oz) black beans, drained and rinsed
- 1/2 tsp chili powder
- 1/2 tsp cumin
- 1/2 tsp paprika
- 8 small corn tortillas
- 1/4 cup chopped cilantro
- 1/4 cup crumbled queso fresco
- 1 lime, cut into wedges
- 1 Tbsp olive oil
- Salt and pepper to taste

PROCEDURE:

1. Preheat oven to 400°F (204°C).
2. Toss sweet potatoes with olive oil, chili powder, cumin, paprika, salt, and pepper. Spread on a baking sheet and roast for 20 min or until tender.
3. In a skillet, heat black beans until warm.
4. Assemble tacos by dividing sweet potatoes and black beans among tortillas.
5. Top with cilantro, queso fresco, and a squeeze of lime juice.

TIPS:

- Add avocado slices for extra creaminess.
- Use flour tortillas if preferred.

NUTRITIONAL VALUES: Calories: 280, Fat: 7g, Carbs: 44g, Protein: 8g, Sugar: 4g

GRILLED VEGGIE AND HUMMUS WRAP

PREPARATION TIME: 10 min

COOKING TIME: 15 min

MODE OF COOKING: Grilling

SERVINGS: 2

INGREDIENTS:

- 2 whole wheat tortillas
- 1/2 cup hummus
- 1 red bell pepper, sliced
- 1 zucchini, sliced
- 1/2 red onion, sliced
- 1 cup baby spinach
- 1 Tbsp olive oil
- Salt and pepper to taste

PROCEDURE:

1. Preheat grill to medium-high heat.
2. Toss bell pepper, zucchini, and red onion with olive oil, salt, and pepper.
3. Grill vegetables until tender and slightly charred, about 5-7 min per side.
4. Spread hummus evenly on each tortilla.
5. Layer grilled vegetables and spinach on top.

6. Roll up the tortillas tightly and cut in half before serving.

TIPS:

- Add feta cheese for extra flavor.
- Use a panini press for a warm, crispy wrap.

NUTRITIONAL VALUES: Calories: 350, Fat: 15g, Carbs: 40g, Protein: 10g, Sugar: 6g

---

CHICKPEA AND SPINACH STEW

PREPARATION TIME: 10 min

COOKING TIME: 20 min

MODE OF COOKING: Simmering

SERVINGS: 4

INGREDIENTS:

- 1 can (15 oz) chickpeas, drained and rinsed
- 1 can (15 oz) diced tomatoes
- 4 cups fresh spinach
- 1 onion, diced
- 2 cloves garlic, minced
- 1 Tbsp olive oil
- 1 tsp cumin
- 1 tsp paprika
- Salt and pepper to taste

PROCEDURE:

1. Heat olive oil in a large pot over medium heat. Add onion and garlic, sauté until fragrant.
2. Add chickpeas, tomatoes, cumin, paprika, salt, and pepper. Simmer for 15 min.
3. Stir in spinach and cook until wilted.
4. Serve hot.

TIPS:

- Serve with a side of whole grain bread.
- Add a dollop of Greek yogurt for creaminess.

NUTRITIONAL VALUES: Calories: 220, Fat: 8g, Carbs: 30g, Protein: 8g, Sugar: 6g

---

BAKED FALAFEL WITH TZATZIKI SAUCE

PREPARATION TIME: 20 min

COOKING TIME: 25 min

MODE OF COOKING: Baking

SERVINGS: 4

INGREDIENTS:

- 1 can (15 oz) chickpeas, drained and rinsed
- 1/4 cup chopped onion
- 2 cloves garlic, minced
- 1/4 cup fresh parsley, chopped
- 1 tsp cumin
- 1 tsp coriander
- 1/4 cup whole wheat flour
- Salt and pepper to taste
- 1 Tbsp olive oil

Tzatziki Sauce:

- 1 cup Greek yogurt
- 1/2 cucumber, grated
- 1 clove garlic, minced
- 1 Tbsp lemon juice
- 1 Tbsp fresh dill, chopped
- Salt and pepper to taste

PROCEDURE:

1. Preheat oven to 375°F (190°C).

2. In a food processor, combine chickpeas, onion, garlic, parsley, cumin, coriander, salt, and pepper. Pulse until mixture is coarse.

3. Stir in whole wheat flour until well combined.

4. Form mixture into small patties and place on a baking sheet lined with parchment paper.

5. Brush with olive oil and bake for 25 min, flipping halfway through.

6. To make tzatziki sauce, combine Greek yogurt, grated cucumber, garlic, lemon juice, dill, salt, and pepper in a bowl. Mix well.

7. Serve baked falafel with tzatziki sauce.

TIPS:

- Serve in a pita with lettuce and tomatoes.
- Add hot sauce for extra spice.

NUTRITIONAL VALUES: Calories: 300, Fat: 10g, Carbs: 40g, Protein: 12g, Sugar: 4g

---

ASIAN CHICKEN LETTUCE WRAPS

PREPARATION TIME: 10 min

COOKING TIME: 15 min

MODE OF COOKING: Sautéing

SERVINGS: 4

INGREDIENTS:

- 1 lb ground chicken
- 1/2 cup diced bell peppers
- 1/2 cup diced carrots
- 1/4 cup diced onions
- 2 cloves garlic, minced
- 1 Tbsp olive oil
- 2 Tbsp soy sauce
- 1 Tbsp hoisin sauce
- 1 tsp sesame oil
- 1 head butter lettuce, leaves separated
- Salt and pepper to taste

PROCEDURE:

1. Heat olive oil in a skillet over medium heat. Add garlic and onions, sauté until fragrant.

2. Add ground chicken and cook until browned.

3. Stir in bell peppers, carrots, soy sauce, hoisin sauce, sesame oil, salt, and pepper. Cook until vegetables are tender.

4. Serve chicken mixture in lettuce leaves.

TIPS:

- Top with chopped peanuts for extra crunch.
- Add a squeeze of lime juice for freshness.

NUTRITIONAL VALUES: Calories: 280, Fat: 14g, Carbs: 10g, Protein: 28g, Sugar: 4g

CAULIFLOWER RICE BURRITO BOWL

PREPARATION TIME: 15 min

COOKING TIME: 10 min

MODE OF COOKING: Sautéing

SERVINGS: 2

INGREDIENTS:

- 1 head cauliflower, riced
- 1 can (15 oz) black beans, drained and rinsed
- 1 cup corn kernels
- 1/2 cup diced tomatoes
- 1/2 cup diced onions
- 1 avocado, sliced
- 1 Tbsp olive oil
- 1 tsp cumin
- 1 tsp chili powder
- Salt and pepper to taste

PROCEDURE:

1. Heat olive oil in a large skillet over medium heat. Add onions and sauté until tender.
2. Add rice cauliflower, cumin, chili powder, salt, and pepper. Cook until cauliflower is tender.
3. In bowls, layer cauliflower rice, black beans, corn, tomatoes, and avocado slices.

TIPS:

- Top with a dollop of Greek yogurt or salsa.
- Add grilled chicken or shrimp for extra protein.

NUTRITIONAL VALUES: Calories: 280, Fat: 14g, Carbs: 34g, Protein: 8g, Sugar: 4g

SPAGHETTI SQUASH WITH MARINARA SAUCE

PREPARATION TIME: 10 min

COOKING TIME: 40 min

MODE OF COOKING: Baking

SERVINGS: 2

INGREDIENTS:

- 1 medium spaghetti squash
- 2 cups marinara sauce
- 1/4 cup grated Parmesan cheese
- 1 Tbsp olive oil
- 2 cloves garlic, minced
- Salt and pepper to taste

PROCEDURE:

1. Preheat oven to 400°F (204°C).
2. Cut spaghetti squash in half lengthwise and remove seeds. Brush with olive oil, season with salt and pepper.
3. Place squash halves cut side down on a baking sheet. Bake for 40 min or until tender.
4. In a saucepan, heat marinara sauce with garlic.
5. Use a fork to scrape out the flesh of the squash into strands. Divide between plates.
6. Top with marinara sauce and sprinkle with Parmesan cheese.

TIPS:

- Add sautéed mushrooms or ground turkey to the sauce.

- Serve with a side salad for a complete meal.

NUTRITIONAL VALUES: Calories: 220, Fat: 10g, Carbs: 28g, Protein: 8g, Sugar: 10g

CHAPTER 5: DINNER RECIPES

LEMON HERB BAKED SALMON

PREPARATION TIME: 10 min

COOKING TIME: 20 min

MODE OF COOKING: Baking

SERVINGS: 4

INGREDIENTS:

- 4 salmon fillets
- 2 Tbsp olive oil
- 1 lemon, thinly sliced
- 2 cloves garlic, minced
- 1 Tbsp fresh dill, chopped
- 1 Tbsp fresh parsley, chopped
- Salt and pepper to taste

PROCEDURE:

1. Preheat oven to 375°F (190°C).
2. Place salmon fillets on a baking sheet lined with parchment paper.
3. Drizzle olive oil over the salmon and season with garlic, dill, parsley, salt, and pepper.
4. Place lemon slices on top of each fillet.
5. Bake for 20 min, or until the salmon is cooked through and flakes easily with a fork.

TIPS:

- Serve with a side of roasted vegetables or a fresh salad.
- Add a splash of white wine for extra flavor.

NUTRITIONAL VALUES: Calories: 350, Fat: 20g, Carbs: 2g, Protein: 35g, Sugar: 0g

QUINOA AND VEGGIE STUFFED BELL PEPPERS

PREPARATION TIME: 15 min

COOKING TIME: 30 min

MODE OF COOKING: Baking

SERVINGS: 4

INGREDIENTS:

- 4 large bell peppers, tops cut off and seeds removed
- 1 cup cooked quinoa
- 1 cup black beans, drained and rinsed
- 1 cup corn kernels
- 1/2 cup diced tomatoes
- 1/4 cup diced red onion
- 1/4 cup shredded cheddar cheese
- 1 tsp cumin
- 1 tsp chili powder
- Salt and pepper to taste

PROCEDURE:

1. Preheat oven to 375°F (190°C).
2. In a bowl, mix cooked quinoa, black beans, corn, tomatoes, onion, cumin, chili powder, salt, and pepper.
3. Stuff each bell pepper with the quinoa mixture.
4. Place stuffed peppers in a baking dish and sprinkle with cheddar cheese.
5. Bake for 30 min, or until the peppers are tender and the cheese is melted.

TIPS:

- Use different colored bell peppers for a vibrant presentation.
- Serve with a dollop of Greek yogurt or salsa.

NUTRITIONAL VALUES: Calories: 300, Fat: 10g, Carbs: 40g, Protein: 12g, Sugar: 6g

---

GRILLED CHICKEN WITH AVOCADO SALSA

PREPARATION TIME: 10 min

COOKING TIME: 15 min

MODE OF COOKING: Grilling

SERVINGS: 4

INGREDIENTS:

- 4 boneless, skinless chicken breasts
- 2 Tbsp olive oil
- 1 tsp garlic powder
- 1 tsp paprika
- 1/2 tsp cumin
- Salt and pepper to taste
- 2 avocados, diced
- 1/2 cup cherry tomatoes, halved
- 1/4 cup red onion, diced
- 1 Tbsp fresh lime juice
- 2 Tbsp fresh cilantro, chopped

PROCEDURE:

1. Preheat grill to medium-high heat.
2. Rub chicken breasts with olive oil, garlic powder, paprika, cumin, salt, and pepper.
3. Grill chicken for 6-7 min per side, or until fully cooked.
4. In a bowl, combine avocados, cherry tomatoes, red onion, lime juice, and cilantro to make the salsa.
5. Serve grilled chicken topped with avocado salsa.

TIPS:

- Serve with a side of quinoa or brown rice.
- Add a squeeze of fresh lime juice for extra flavor.

NUTRITIONAL VALUES: Calories: 320, Fat: 18g, Carbs: 10g, Protein: 32g, Sugar: 1g

---

SPAGHETTI SQUASH PRIMAVERA

PREPARATION TIME: 15 min

COOKING TIME: 40 min

MODE OF COOKING: Baking and Sautéing

SERVINGS: 4

INGREDIENTS:

- 1 large spaghetti squash
- 1 cup cherry tomatoes, halved
- 1 cup zucchini, diced
- 1 cup yellow squash, diced
- 1/2 cup red bell pepper, diced
- 1/4 cup red onion, diced
- 2 cloves garlic, minced
- 2 Tbsp olive oil
- 1/4 cup grated Parmesan cheese
- Salt and pepper to taste

- 1 Tbsp fresh basil, chopped

PROCEDURE:

1. Preheat oven to 400°F (204°C).
2. Cut spaghetti squash in half lengthwise and remove seeds. Brush with olive oil, season with salt and pepper.
3. Place squash halves cut side down on a baking sheet. Bake for 40 min or until tender.
4. In a skillet, heat remaining olive oil over medium heat. Add garlic and onion, sauté until fragrant.
5. Add cherry tomatoes, zucchini, yellow squash, and red bell pepper. Cook until tender.
6. Use a fork to scrape out the flesh of the squash into strands and add to the skillet.
7. Toss with vegetables, season with salt and pepper, and sprinkle with Parmesan cheese and fresh basil.

TIPS:

- Serve with a side of garlic bread.
- Add cooked chicken or shrimp for extra protein.

NUTRITIONAL VALUES: Calories: 250, Fat: 12g, Carbs: 28g, Protein: 7g, Sugar: 8g

---

BEEF AND BROCCOLI STIR-FRY

PREPARATION TIME: 10 min
COOKING TIME: 15 min
MODE OF COOKING: Sautéing
SERVINGS: 4
INGREDIENTS:

- 1 lb beef sirloin, thinly sliced
- 3 cups broccoli florets
- 1 red bell pepper, sliced
- 2 cloves garlic, minced
- 1 Tbsp fresh ginger, grated
- 3 Tbsp soy sauce
- 1 Tbsp oyster sauce
- 1 Tbsp cornstarch
- 1 Tbsp sesame oil
- 1 Tbsp olive oil
- 1/4 cup water
- 1 tsp sesame seeds (optional)

PROCEDURE:

1. In a bowl, toss beef with cornstarch until well coated.
2. Heat olive oil in a large skillet over medium-high heat. Add beef and cook until browned, about 3-4 min. Remove from skillet and set aside.
3. In the same skillet, add sesame oil, garlic, and ginger. Sauté until fragrant.
4. Add broccoli and red bell pepper, stir-fry for 5 min.
5. Return beef to the skillet and add soy sauce, oyster sauce, and water. Cook for another 3-4 min until everything is well coated and heated through.
6. Sprinkle with sesame seeds before serving.

- Serve over steamed rice or noodles.
- Add a splash of sriracha for a spicy kick.

NUTRITIONAL VALUES: Calories: 350, Fat: 18g, Carbs: 18g, Protein: 28g, Sugar: 4g

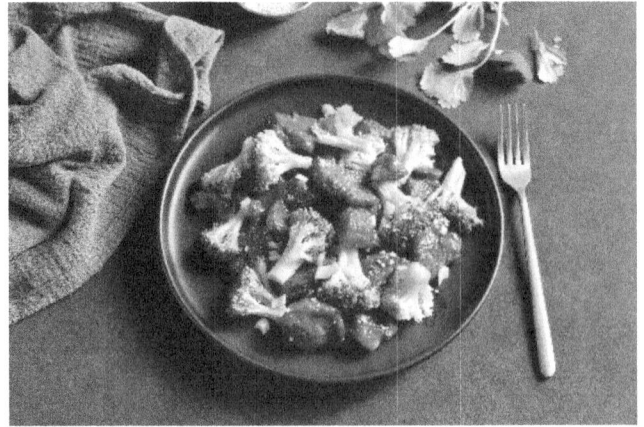

CHICKEN AND SPINACH STUFFED SWEET POTATOES

PREPARATION TIME: 15 min

COOKING TIME: 45 min

MODE OF COOKING: Baking

SERVINGS: 4

INGREDIENTS:

- 4 medium sweet potatoes
- 2 cups cooked, shredded chicken breast
- 2 cups fresh spinach
- 1/2 cup Greek yogurt
- 1/4 cup shredded mozzarella cheese
- 2 cloves garlic, minced
- 1 Tbsp olive oil
- Salt and pepper to taste

PROCEDURE:

1. Preheat oven to 375°F (190°C).
2. Wash sweet potatoes and pierce with a fork. Bake for 45 min or until tender.
3. In a skillet, heat olive oil over medium heat. Add garlic and spinach, cook until wilted.
4. In a bowl, mix shredded chicken, cooked spinach, Greek yogurt, salt, and pepper.
5. Once sweet potatoes are done, cut them in half and scoop out a portion of the flesh to create a well.
6. Stuff the sweet potatoes with the chicken mixture and sprinkle with mozzarella cheese.
7. Return to the oven for 10 min or until cheese is melted.

TIPS:

- Serve with a side salad for a complete meal.
- Add hot sauce for extra flavor.

NUTRITIONAL VALUES: Calories: 380, Fat: 12g, Carbs: 42g, Protein: 28g, Sugar: 12g

BAKED COD WITH GARLIC AND HERBS

PREPARATION TIME: 10 min

COOKING TIME: 20 min

MODE OF COOKING: Baking

SERVINGS: 4

INGREDIENTS:

- 4 cod fillets
- 2 Tbsp olive oil
- 2 cloves garlic, minced
- 1 lemon, zested and juiced
- 1 Tbsp fresh parsley, chopped
- 1 tsp dried thyme
- Salt and pepper to taste

PROCEDURE:

1. Preheat oven to 400°F (204°C).
2. Place cod fillets in a baking dish. Drizzle with olive oil and lemon juice.
3. In a small bowl, mix garlic, lemon zest, parsley, thyme, salt, and pepper. Spread over the cod fillets.
4. Bake for 20 min or until the fish is opaque and flakes easily with a fork.

TIPS:

- Serve with steamed vegetables or a side of quinoa.
- Add a sprinkle of Parmesan cheese for extra flavor.

NUTRITIONAL VALUES: Calories: 220, Fat: 10g, Carbs: 2g, Protein: 30g, Sugar: 0g

VEGETARIAN STUFFED PORTOBELLO MUSHROOMS

PREPARATION TIME: 15 min

COOKING TIME: 25 min

MODE OF COOKING: Baking

SERVINGS: 4

INGREDIENTS:

- 4 large portobello mushrooms, stems removed
- 1 cup cooked quinoa
- 1 cup spinach, chopped
- 1/2 cup cherry tomatoes, diced
- 1/4 cup feta cheese, crumbled
- 2 cloves garlic, minced
- 1 Tbsp olive oil
- Salt and pepper to taste

PROCEDURE:

1. Preheat oven to 375°F (190°C).
2. Brush mushrooms with olive oil and place on a baking sheet.
3. In a bowl, mix quinoa, spinach, cherry tomatoes, feta cheese, garlic, salt, and pepper.
4. Stuff each mushroom with the quinoa mixture.
5. Bake for 25 min or until mushrooms are tender and filling is heated through.

TIPS:

- Serve with a side of mixed greens.
- Add a sprinkle of pine nuts for added texture.

NUTRITIONAL VALUES: Calories: 250, Fat: 12g, Carbs: 24g, Protein: 10g, Sugar: 4g

TURKEY AND ZUCCHINI MEATBALLS

PREPARATION TIME: 15 min

COOKING TIME: 25 min

MODE OF COOKING: Baking

SERVINGS: 4

INGREDIENTS:

- 1 lb ground turkey
- 1 cup grated zucchini
- 1/4 cup breadcrumbs
- 1 egg
- 2 cloves garlic, minced
- 1 tsp dried oregano
- 1 tsp dried basil
- Salt and pepper to taste
- 1 Tbsp olive oil

PROCEDURE:

1. Preheat oven to 400°F (204°C).

2. In a bowl, combine ground turkey, grated zucchini, breadcrumbs, egg, garlic, oregano, basil, salt, and pepper. Mix well.

3. Form mixture into meatballs and place on a baking sheet lined with parchment paper.

4. Drizzle with olive oil and bake for 25 min or until meatballs are cooked through.

TIPS:

- Serve with marinara sauce over whole wheat pasta.
- Add a sprinkle of Parmesan cheese before serving.

NUTRITIONAL VALUES: Calories: 300, Fat: 18g, Carbs: 10g, Protein: 25g, Sugar: 2g

SHRIMP AND ASPARAGUS STIR-FRY

PREPARATION TIME: 10 min

COOKING TIME: 10 min

MODE OF COOKING: Sautéing

SERVINGS: 4

INGREDIENTS:

- 1 lb shrimp, peeled and deveined
- 1 bunch asparagus, trimmed and cut into 2-inch pieces
- 1 red bell pepper, sliced
- 2 cloves garlic, minced
- 1 Tbsp fresh ginger, grated
- 2 Tbsp soy sauce
- 1 Tbsp hoisin sauce
- 1 tsp sesame oil
- 1 Tbsp olive oil
- Salt and pepper to taste

PROCEDURE:

1. Heat olive oil in a large skillet over medium-high heat. Add garlic and ginger, sauté until fragrant.

2. Add shrimp and cook until pink and opaque, about 3-4 min. Remove from skillet and set aside.

3. In the same skillet, add asparagus and red bell pepper. Stir-fry until tender.

4. Return shrimp to the skillet and add soy sauce, hoisin sauce, sesame oil,

salt, and pepper. Cook for another 2-3 min until everything is well coated and heated through.

TIPS:

- Serve over steamed rice or noodles.
- Add red pepper flakes for a spicy kick.

NUTRITIONAL VALUES: Calories: 250, Fat: 10g, Carbs: 12g, Protein: 28g, Sugar: 4g

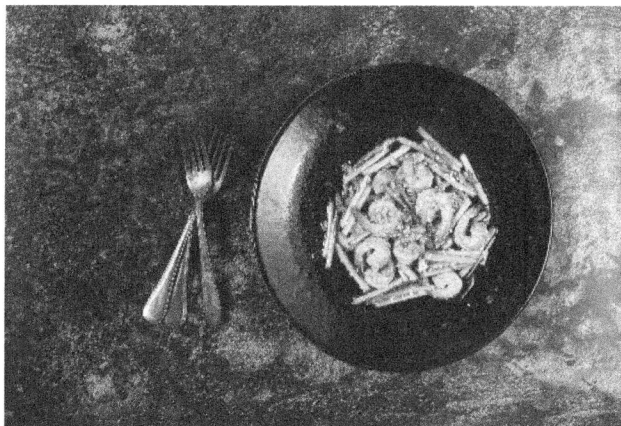

CHICKEN AND BROCCOLI ALFREDO

PREPARATION TIME: 15 min

COOKING TIME: 20 min

MODE OF COOKING: Sautéing

SERVINGS: 4

INGREDIENTS:

- 2 boneless, skinless chicken breasts, sliced
- 2 cups broccoli florets
- 1 cup low-fat milk
- 1/2 cup grated Parmesan cheese
- 2 cloves garlic, minced
- 2 Tbsp olive oil
- 2 Tbsp flour
- 1/2 tsp salt
- 1/4 tsp black pepper
- 8 oz whole wheat pasta

PROCEDURE:

1. Cook pasta according to package instructions. Drain and set aside.
2. In a large skillet, heat olive oil over medium heat. Add chicken and cook until browned and cooked through. Remove from skillet and set aside.
3. In the same skillet, add garlic and cook until fragrant. Add flour and cook for 1 min.
4. Gradually whisk in milk, stirring constantly until the sauce thickens.
5. Stir in Parmesan cheese, salt, and pepper.
6. Add broccoli and cooked chicken to the sauce. Cook until broccoli is tender.
7. Toss in the cooked pasta and mix well.

TIPS:

- Use cauliflower instead of broccoli for a different twist.
- Add red pepper flakes for a spicy kick.

NUTRITIONAL VALUES: Calories: 400, Fat: 15g, Carbs: 42g, Protein: 28g, Sugar: 3g

MAPLE GLAZED SALMON

PREPARATION TIME: 10 min

COOKING TIME: 20 min

MODE OF COOKING: Baking

SERVINGS: 4

INGREDIENTS:

- 4 salmon fillets
- 1/4 cup pure maple syrup
- 2 Tbsp soy sauce
- 1 Tbsp Dijon mustard
- 2 cloves garlic, minced
- Salt and pepper to taste

PROCEDURE:

1. Preheat oven to 400°F (204°C).
2. In a small bowl, whisk together maple syrup, soy sauce, Dijon mustard, garlic, salt, and pepper.
3. Place salmon fillets in a baking dish and pour the maple glaze over them.
4. Bake for 20 min or until the salmon is cooked through and flakes easily with a fork.

TIPS:

- Serve with a side of steamed vegetables or quinoa.
- Garnish with chopped parsley for extra freshness.

NUTRITIONAL VALUES: Calories: 320, Fat: 14g, Carbs: 18g, Protein: 28g, Sugar: 15g

BEEF AND VEGETABLE STIR-FRY

PREPARATION TIME: 10 min

COOKING TIME: 15 min

MODE OF COOKING: Sautéing

SERVINGS: 4

INGREDIENTS:

- 1 lb beef sirloin, thinly sliced
- 2 cups broccoli florets
- 1 red bell pepper, sliced
- 1 cup snap peas
- 1/2 cup sliced carrots
- 2 cloves garlic, minced
- 2 Tbsp soy sauce
- 1 Tbsp hoisin sauce
- 1 tsp sesame oil
- 1 Tbsp olive oil
- Salt and pepper to taste

PROCEDURE:

1. Heat olive oil in a large skillet over medium-high heat. Add beef and cook until browned. Remove from skillet and set aside.
2. In the same skillet, add garlic and cook until fragrant.
3. Add broccoli, bell pepper, snap peas, and carrots. Stir-fry until vegetables are tender.
4. Return beef to the skillet and add soy sauce, hoisin sauce, sesame oil, salt, and pepper. Cook for another 2-3 min until everything is well coated and heated through.

TIPS:

- Serve over steamed rice or noodles.
- Add red pepper flakes for a spicy kick.

NUTRITIONAL VALUES: Calories: 350, Fat: 18g, Carbs: 18g, Protein: 28g, Sugar: 4g

---

LEMON GARLIC SHRIMP PASTA

PREPARATION TIME: 10 min

COOKING TIME: 20 min

MODE OF COOKING: Sautéing

SERVINGS: 4

INGREDIENTS:

- 12 oz whole wheat pasta
- 1 lb shrimp, peeled and deveined
- 4 cloves garlic, minced
- 1/4 cup olive oil
- 1/4 cup fresh lemon juice
- 1/4 cup grated Parmesan cheese
- 1/4 cup chopped fresh parsley
- Salt and pepper to taste

PROCEDURE:

1. Cook pasta according to package instructions. Drain and set aside.
2. In a large skillet, heat olive oil over medium heat. Add garlic and cook until fragrant.
3. Add shrimp and cook until pink and opaque, about 3-4 min.
4. Stir in lemon juice, Parmesan cheese, salt, and pepper.
5. Add cooked pasta to the skillet and toss to combine.
6. Sprinkle with fresh parsley before serving.

TIPS:

- Add red pepper flakes for a spicy kick.
- Serve with a side of garlic bread.

NUTRITIONAL VALUES: Calories: 400, Fat: 18g, Carbs: 42g, Protein: 28g, Sugar: 3g

---

CHICKEN FAJITA BOWL

PREPARATION TIME: 15 min

COOKING TIME: 20 min

MODE OF COOKING: Sautéing

SERVINGS: 4

INGREDIENTS:

- 2 boneless, skinless chicken breasts, sliced
- 1 red bell pepper, sliced
- 1 green bell pepper, sliced
- 1 yellow bell pepper, sliced
- 1 onion, sliced
- 2 cloves garlic, minced
- 2 Tbsp olive oil
- 1 tsp cumin
- 1 tsp chili powder
- 1/2 tsp paprika
- Salt and pepper to taste
- 2 cups cooked brown rice
- 1 avocado, sliced
- 1/4 cup chopped cilantro

PROCEDURE:

1. Heat olive oil in a large skillet over

medium-high heat. Add garlic and cook until fragrant.

2. Add chicken and cook until browned and cooked through.

3. Add bell peppers, onion, cumin, chili powder, paprika, salt, and pepper. Cook until vegetables are tender.

4. Divide cooked brown rice between bowls and top with the chicken and vegetable mixture.

5. Garnish with avocado slices and chopped cilantro.

TIPS:

- Serve with a side of salsa or Greek yogurt.
- Add black beans for extra protein.

NUTRITIONAL VALUES: Calories: 450, Fat: 20g, Carbs: 42g, Protein: 28g, Sugar: 4g

TURKEY MEATLOAF

PREPARATION TIME: 15 min

COOKING TIME: 45 min

MODE OF COOKING: Baking

SERVINGS: 4

INGREDIENTS:

- 1 lb ground turkey
- 1/2 cup breadcrumbs
- 1/2 cup finely chopped onion
- 1/4 cup milk
- 1 egg
- 2 cloves garlic, minced
- 1 Tbsp Worcestershire sauce
- 1 tsp dried thyme
- 1 tsp dried oregano
- Salt and pepper to taste
- 1/4 cup ketchup

PROCEDURE:

1. Preheat oven to 375°F (190°C).

2. In a large bowl, combine ground turkey, breadcrumbs, onion, milk, egg, garlic, Worcestershire sauce, thyme, oregano, salt, and pepper. Mix well.

3. Shape the mixture into a loaf and place in a baking dish.

4. Spread ketchup over the top of the meatloaf.

5. Bake for 45 min or until the meatloaf is cooked through.

TIPS:

- Serve with mashed potatoes or steamed vegetables.
- Add a splash of hot sauce for extra flavor.

NUTRITIONAL VALUES: Calories: 300, Fat: 10g, Carbs: 20g, Protein: 28g, Sugar: 6g

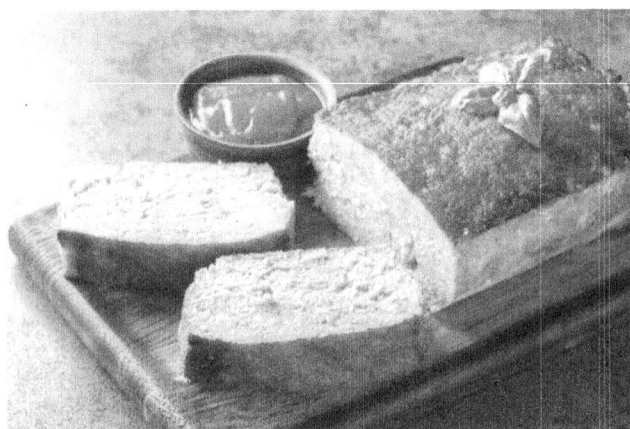

SPAGHETTI BOLOGNESE

PREPARATION TIME: 15 min

COOKING TIME: 30 min

MODE OF COOKING: Sautéing and Simmering

SERVINGS: 4

INGREDIENTS:

- 12 oz whole wheat spaghetti
- 1 lb lean ground beef
- 1 onion, diced
- 2 cloves garlic, minced
- 1 can (28 oz) crushed tomatoes
- 1/4 cup tomato paste
- 1/2 cup red wine (optional)
- 1 tsp dried oregano
- 1 tsp dried basil
- 1/4 tsp red pepper flakes
- 2 Tbsp olive oil
- Salt and pepper to taste
- 1/4 cup grated Parmesan cheese

PROCEDURE:

1. Cook spaghetti according to package instructions. Drain and set aside.
2. In a large skillet, heat olive oil over medium heat. Add onion and garlic, cook until fragrant.
3. Add ground beef and cook until browned.
4. Stir in crushed tomatoes, tomato paste, red wine (if using), oregano, basil, red pepper flakes, salt, and pepper. Simmer for 20 min.
5. Serve the sauce over cooked spaghetti and sprinkle with Parmesan cheese.

TIPS:

- Serve with a side salad and garlic bread.
- Use ground turkey or chicken for a lighter option.

NUTRITIONAL VALUES: Calories: 450, Fat: 18g, Carbs: 48g, Protein: 28g, Sugar: 6g

CHAPTER 6: 30-DAY MEAL PLAN

WEEK 1-2	breakfast	snack	lunch	snack	dinner
Monday	Oatmeal with Blueberries	Sliced apple	Grilled Chicken Salad	Greek yogurt	Baked Salmon with Asparagus
Tuesday	Scrambled Eggs with Spinach	Celery sticks with peanut butter	Quinoa and Black Bean Salad	Carrot sticks	Turkey Meatballs with Zoodles
Wednesday	Smoothie with Banana and Almond Milk	Mixed nuts	Chicken Caesar Salad	Sliced bell peppers	Grilled Shrimp and Veggie Skewers
Thursday	Greek Yogurt with Honey and Walnuts	Fresh berries	Tuna Salad Lettuce Wraps	A small handful of almonds	Stuffed Bell Peppers
Friday	Avocado Toast with Poached Egg	Cucumber slices	Lentil Soup	A small orange	Baked Cod with Broccoli
Saturday	Cottage Cheese with Pineapple	Sliced pear	Spinach and Feta Salad	Cherry tomatoes	Chicken Stir Fry
Sunday	Whole Grain Pancakes with Maple Syrup	Baby carrots	Chickpea Salad	A handful of grapes	Beef and Vegetable Stew

WEEK 3-4	breakfast	snack	lunch	snack	dinner
Monday	Chia Pudding with Mango	Carrot sticks	Turkey and Avocado Wrap	Greek yogurt	Grilled Swordfish with Vegetables
Tuesday	Egg Muffins with Vegetables	Sliced pear	Greek Salad with Quinoa	A handful of almonds	Spaghetti Squash with Marinara Sauce
Wednesday	Berry Smoothie with Spinach	Sliced cucumber	Cobb Salad	Baby carrots	Lemon Herb Chicken with Green Beans
Thursday	Overnight Oats with Chia Seeds	Sliced apple	Vegetable Soup	Sliced bell peppers	Grilled Pork Chops with Apples
Friday	Whole Wheat Toast with Almond Butter	Mixed berries	Salmon Salad	A handful of walnuts	Shrimp Stir Fry with Broccoli
Saturday	Banana Pancakes	Sliced kiwi	Caprese Salad	Greek yogurt	Stuffed Zucchini Boats
Sunday	Yogurt Parfait with Granola	Sliced bell peppers	Black Bean Soup	A handful of grapes	Beef Stir Fry with Mixed Veggies

MEASUREMENT CONVERSION TABLE

Volume Conversions

Volume (Liquid)	US Customary Units	Metric Units
1 teaspoon	1 tsp	5 milliliters (ml)
1 tablespoon	1 tbsp	15 milliliters
1 fluid ounce	1 fl oz	30 milliliters
1 cup	1 cup	240 milliliters
1 pint	1 pt	473 milliliters
1 quart	1 qt	946 milliliters
1 gallon	1 gal	3.785 liters

Weight Conversions

Weight	US Customary Units	Metric Units
1 ounce	1 oz	28 grams (g)
1 pound	1 lb	454 grams
1 kilogram	2.2 lbs	1000 grams (1 kg)

Length Conversions

Length	US Customary Units	Metric Units
1 inch	1 in	2.54 centimeters (cm)
1 foot	1 ft	30.48 centimeters

Metric Volume Conversions

Volume	Metric Units	US Customary Units
1 milliliter (ml)	1 ml	0.034 fluid ounce (fl oz)
100 milliliters	100 ml	3.4 fluid ounces
1 liter (L)	1 L	34 fluid ounces
		4.2 cups
		2.1 pints

Volume	Metric Units	US Customary Units
		1.06 quarts
		0.26 gallon

Metric Weight Conversions

Weight	Metric Units	US Customary Units
1 gram (g)	1 g	0.035 ounces (oz)
100 grams	100 g	3.5 ounces
500 grams	500 g	1.1 pounds (lb)
1 kilogram (kg)	1 kg	2.2 pounds

Temperature Conversions

Temperature	Celsius (°C)	Fahrenheit (°F)
Freezing Point	0°C	32°F
Refrigerator	4°C	39°F
Room Temperature	20°C - 22°C	68°F - 72°F
Boiling Water	100°C	212°F

CHAPTER 7: SUCCESS STORIES FROM DR. NOWZARADAN'S PATIENTS

Success in any endeavor is best illuminated through stories of real people who have walked the path and seen significant transformations. The 1200-calorie diet plan developed by Dr. Nowzaradan has not just been a theoretical exercise in nutrition but a practical lifesaver for many of his patients. The narratives of these individuals don't merely chart a course of losing weight; they tell of regained lives, restored health, and renewed hope.

Sarah, a 34-year-old elementary school teacher from Texas, had reached a point where her weight affected both her professional life and personal self-esteem. With a busy schedule filled with managing classrooms and after-school programs, Sarah had little time to invest in lengthy meal preparations or elaborate fitness routines. Her journey with Dr. Nowzaradan's diet plan began reluctantly, underscored by previous failures that made her skeptical. However, what differentiated this plan for Sarah was its simplicity and direct approach. Within the first month, by adhering strictly to the 1200-calorie regime and simple, quick recipes, Sarah lost 12 pounds. It wasn't just the weight loss, but the surge in her energy levels and ability to participate in activities with her students that marked the early success of her dieting efforts.

Mark's story is one of psychological triumph as much as it is about physical transformation. At 45, and after two decades spent in a sedentary job, Mark's health metrics were pointing him towards serious risks of diabetes and cardiovascular diseases. Mark's journey began on a somber note when a close friend suffered a heart attack, a life event that mirrored his own health trajectory. Dr. Nowzaradan's plan for Mark was more than a diet; it was a wakeup call. Over six months, not only did Mark significantly reduce his weight by following the 1200-calorie guideline, but his regular consultations with Dr. Nowzaradan also educated him on the permanent dietary adjustments needed to sustain his healthier lifestyle. His success story is shared often by Dr. Now, highlighting the psychological attitude adjustment toward food and health that is essential for long-term success. Jenna and Tom, a couple in their late 30s, embarked on the 1200-calorie diet journey together after years of unsuccessful attempts at dieting separately. Their partnership in this health endeavor provided a support system that was crucial in overcoming the dieting challenges. With specific adaptations to the diet plan that catered to each of their tastes and health requirements, they not only cheered each other through plateaus and celebrated each pound lost but also found a renewed connection in their relationship. Their story stresses the aspect of community and support in Dr. Nowzaradan's approach, demonstrating that sometimes, the path to personal health can be a joint venture.

Elena, a retiree and grandmother from North Carolina, shows that it is never too late to start on a path to healthier living. Before starting Dr. Nowzaradan's diet, Elena had accepted poor health as a part of aging. However, post a worrying doctor's visit where she was confronted with the possibility of imminent invasive surgeries due to her weight and related complications, Elena decided to take charge. Her manipulation of the 1200-calorie plan to fit her dietary restrictions due to older age and her dedication to following through with the diet's requirements despite initial difficulties is a testament to her strength. Six months later, not only did she forego the need for medical interventions, but she also took up gardening, an activity she thought she had left behind in her younger years.

Dr. Nowzaradan often points out that the effectiveness of his 1200-calorie diet plan is evidenced not just in physical weight loss but in the overall enhancement of quality of life, as shown by these patients. Sarah, Mark, Jenna, Tom, and Elena represent countless others who have found significant life changes through this program. They illustrate that while the diet is structured and rigorous, it is flexible enough to be adapted to individual needs and situations, promoting a sustainable lifestyle shift that prioritizes long-term health over short-term gains.

Through these stories of genuine experiences, it becomes clear that Dr. Nowzaradan's 1200-calorie diet is more than a regime—it's a doorway to reclaiming a healthier, more engaged life. Each story is unique, yet they all converge on common themes of overcoming initial doubts, the importance of consistency, and the transformative power of adopting a healthy eating lifestyle.

These narratives are crucial for new participants in the diet plan, providing them not just with hope, but also with practical illustrations of how they might similarly address their challenges. The success stories from Dr. Nowzaradan's patients underscore the profound impact that well-informed and carefully guided dietary planning can have on individual lives. They serve not only as testimonials to the effectiveness of the 1200-calorie diet but also as motivational beacons for others embarking on similar journeys. The path to health is often riddled with challenges, but as these stories show, the journey and its rewards are well worth the effort.

CHAPTER 8: CONCLUSION

As we reach the conclusion of this guided journey through Dr. Nowzaradan's 1200-Calorie Diet Plan, it's essential to reflect on what we've learned and the transformative potential this plan holds for your life. We've traversed from understanding the robust scientific foundations that underscore the necessity and effectiveness of a controlled calorie intake, to the practical application of these principles through meal plans and inspiring recipes. It's been a journey not just about weight loss but about gaining a deeper understanding of health and how our bodies respond to what we feed them.

From the early chapters, where we explored Dr. Nowzaradan's philosophy and the scientific bedrock of rapid weight loss, to the succeeding sections laden with nutritious recipes, it becomes clear that every element of this diet plan has been crafted with two things in mind: sustainability and health enhancement. In adopting this Diet Plan, you weren't just handed a set of rules to follow; you were provided a framework to understand your body's needs and how to address them thoughtfully.

Dieting, especially in a world filled with quick fixes and flashy health fads, can often lead to a disconnection from the reality of what truly works. Through your adherence to the 1200-calorie diet, however, you've been connected with a fundamental truth: health transformation requires dedication, understanding, and adaptability. Whether it's adjusting portion sizes, substituting ingredients to suit your metabolic needs, or pacing your meals to keep hunger at bay, the adaptability of this diet speaks to its robust foundation.

One of the most heartening aspects captured in this book is the stories of individuals who, like you, embarked on this journey often laden with skepticism but emerged not only lighter in weight but also enriched in a lifestyle that promotes vitality. Their testimonies aren't just stories of weight loss; they are narratives of regained confidence, improved mobility, and reclaimed lives. These stories underscore a critical aspect of the Dr. Now Diet Plan: it is not a temporary regimen but a gateway to a renewed, sustainable way of living.

Moreover, as evidenced by the scientific discussions and the detailed explanation of macronutrients and micronutrients, Dr. Nowzaradan's diet plan transcends the mere act of eating less. It's about understanding what you eat, how it affects your body, and how you can manage these implications to foster overall well-being. The discussions about metabolism and the role of various nutrients in your body were aimed at equipping you with knowledge that anchors your daily dietary choices in science, not trends.

As you move forward, it's important to carry with you not just the recipes or the specific guidelines but the principles that they embody. Maintain the curiosity about how foods affect your body, keep assessing and adjusting as your health evolves, and hold onto the understanding that eating is an integral part of life's balance. The essentials of portion control, the significance of regular meal tracking, and the strategies to handle social pressures while sticking to your diet are all tools designed to empower you, giving you control over your health destiny.

Now, as you close this book and perhaps begin to write the next chapter of your health journey, remember that every small change you have implemented is a building block for a stronger foundation of health. Whether it's choosing a protein-rich breakfast to kickstart your metabolism or wisely navigating a dinner menu at a family gathering, each decision is a testament to your commitment to live a healthier, fuller life.

Lastly, let's acknowledge that while diet is a monumental factor in health, it works best when complemented by other lifestyle adjustments, including regular physical activity and mental health management. Treat this diet plan as a part of a holistic approach to health. Take walks, practice mindfulness, connect with supportive communities, and never hesitate to seek professional guidance when you feel stuck.

Remember, the journey to weight loss and improved health is not linear. It comes with its up and downs, its challenges and triumphs. Armed with the knowledge from Dr. Nowzaradan's 1200-Calorie Diet Plan, plus your experiences and the community's support, you are better equipped to navigate this journey.

Continue to live with the awareness and discipline that you've cultivated through this program, and let each meal be a reflection of not just your health goals but also your newfound respect for nourishment and wellbeing. Here's to your health, your energy, and a vibrant life ahead.

Made in the USA
Las Vegas, NV
02 February 2025